D1252357

Antibiotic Use in Dermatology

Guest Editor

JAMES Q. DEL ROSSO, DO, FAOCD

DERMATOLOGIC CLINICS

www.derm.theclinics.com

Consulting Editor
BRUCE H. THIERS, MD

January 2009 • Volume 27 • Number 1

SAUNDERS an imprint of ELSEVIER, Inc.

W.B. SAUNDERS COMPANY
A Division of Elsevier Inc.

1600 John F. Kennedy Boulevard • Suite 1800 • Philadelphia, PA 19103-2899

http://www.theclinics.com

DERMATOLOGIC CLINICS Volume 27, Number 1
January 2009 ISSN 0733-8635, ISBN-13: 978-1-4377-0468-6, ISBN 10: 1-4377-0468-9

Editor: Carla Holloway
Developmental Editor: Donald Mumford

Dermatologic Clinics (ISSN 0733-8635) is published quarterly by Elsevier Inc., 360 Park Avenue South, New York, NY 10010-1710. Months of publication are January, April, July, and October. Business and editorial offices: 1600 John F. Kennedy Blvd., Suite 1800, Philadelphia, PA 19103-2899. Customer service office: 11830 Westline Drive, St. Louis, MO 63146. Periodicals postage paid at New York, NY, and additional mailing offices. Subscription prices are USD 274.00 per year for US individuals, USD 423.00 per year for US institutions, USD 321.00 per year for Canadian individuals, USD 506.00 per year for Canadian institutions, USD 376.00 per year for international individuals, USD 506.00 per year for international institutions, USD 131.00 per year for US students/residents, and USD 189.00 per year for Canadian and international students/residents. International air speed delivery is included in all *Clinics* subscription prices. All prices are subject to change without notice. **POSTMASTER:** Send address changes to *Dermatologic Clinics*, Elsevier Journals Customer Service, 11830 Westline Drive, St. Louis, MO 63146. **Customer Service: 1-800-654-2452 (US and Canada). From outside of the US and Canada, call 1-314-453-7041. Fax: 1-314-453-5170. For print support, e-mail: JournalsCustomer Service-usa@elsevier.com. For online support, e-mail: JournalsOnlineSupport-usa@elsevier.com.**

Reprints. For copies of 100 or more, of articles in this publication, please contact the Commercial Reprints Department, Elsevier Inc., 360 Park Avenue South, New York, New York 10010-1710. Tel.: (212) 633-3813; Fax: (212) 462-1935; Email: repritns@elsevier.com.

The *Dermatologic Clinics* is covered in *MEDLINE/PubMed (Index Medicus)*, *Current Contents/Clinical Medicine*, *Excerpta Medica*, *Chemical Abstracts*, and *ISI/BIOMED*.

Printed in the United States of America.

Contributors

GUEST EDITOR

JAMES Q. DEL ROSSO, DO, FAOCD
Dermatology Residency Director, Valley Hospital
Medical Center, Las Vegas, Nevada

AUTHORS

AVANI BHAMBRI, MD
Dermatology Resident, University of California
Los Angeles Medical Center, Los Angeles,
California

SANJAY BHAMBRI, DO
Chief Resident, Dermatology Valley Hospital
Medical Center, Las Vegas, Nevada

NEAL BHATIA, MD
Associate Clinical Professor, University
of Wisconsin, Madison, Wisconsin

JAMES Q. DEL ROSSO, DO, FAOCD
Dermatology Residency Director, Valley Hospital
Medical Center, Las Vegas, Nevada

DIRK M. ELSTON, MD
Director, Department of Dermatology, Geisinger
Medical Center, Danville, Pennsylvania

MANDY HARTING, MD
Department of Dermatology, Baylor College
of Medicine; and Dermatology Service, Michael
E. DeBakey Veterans Affairs Medical Center,
Houston, Texas

J.V. HIRSCHMANN, MD
Professor of Medicine, Division of General Internal
Medicine, University of Washington School
of Medicine; and Staff Physician, Medical Service,
Puget Sound Veterans Affairs Medical Center,
Seattle, Washington

GRACE KIM, DO
Valley Hospital Medical Center, Las Vegas,
Nevada

JAMES J. LEYDEN, MD
Emeritus Professor of Dermatology, University
of Pennsylvania, Philadelphia, Pennsylvania

KARL F. POPP, RPh
Independent Consultant and Pharmacist,
Schodack Landing, New York

TED ROSEN, MD
Department of Dermatology, Baylor College
of Medicine; and Dermatology Service, Michael
E. DeBakey Veterans Affairs Medical Center,
Houston, Texas

EMIL A. TANGHETTI, MD
Clinical Professor, Department of Dermatology,
University of California at Davis, Davis; and
Director, Center for Dermatology and Laser
Surgery, Sacramento, California

TRAVIS VANDERGRIFF, MD
Department of Dermatology, Baylor College
of Medicine; and Dermatology Service, Michael
E. DeBakey Veterans Affairs Medical Center,
Houston, Texas

GUY F. WEBSTER, MD, PhD
Department of Dermatology, Jefferson Medical
College, Philadelphia, Pennsylvania

Contents

Clinical Considerations in the Treatment of Acne Vulgaris and Other Inflammatory Skin Disorders: a Status Report   1

James J. Leyden, James Q. Del Rosso, and Guy F. Webster

> This article reviews the anti-inflammatory and nonantimicrobial effects of antibiotics in acne and other diseases and examines issues relating to the emergence of decreased bacterial sensitivity to antibiotics and how these issues relate to clinical practice. It includes an overview of the inflammatory activities of some antibiotic agents and their potential for use in various dermatologic and nondermatologic diseases. It demonstrates that P *acnes*–resistant organisms may be associated with therapeutic failure in some patients with acne, and that the prudent use of antibiotics is necessary to ensure that we can continue to use these drugs to combat disease effectively. It concludes that there are treatment strategies that can effectively minimize the potential for development of resistant P *acnes* organisms.

A Current Review of Topical Benzoyl Peroxide: New Perspectives on Formulation and Utilization   17

Emil A. Tanghetti and Karl F. Popp

> Benzoyl peroxide (BPO) is the most widely used topical acne treatment, with significant antibacterial, antikeratolytic, and comedolytic activity. It has been shown to be extremely effective as monotherapy and in combination with antibiotics or retinoids for managing comedonal and inflammatory acne lesions. As numerous clinical studies have shown, the combination of BPO plus a topical antibiotic is not only more effective but also is often better tolerated than either agent alone. Unlike antibiotics, no bacterial resistance has been noted. Adding BPO to any long-term antibiotic regimen in acne is generally recommended to help reduce populations of drug-resistant variants. Although effective combinations of BPO and antibiotics or retinoids are used, BPO monotherapy can also be extremely effective in treating mild to moderate acne with no resistance issues.

Topical Antibiotics in Dermatology: Emerging Patterns of Resistance   25

Dirk M. Elston

> Resistance to topical antibiotics is increasingly relevant in dermatology. This article discusses emerging patterns of resistance and the implications for clinical practice. Emergence of resistance is complicating decolonization of the skin and nares in patients infected with methicillin-resistant Staphylococcus aureus. In the setting of acne treatment, adding topical benzoyl peroxide has been shown to reduce the emergence of strains resistant to topical antibiotics. Other agents, such as zinc salts, are promising in this regard. This article discusses alternatives to antibiotics and mechanisms to stem the emergence of resistance.

Oral antibiotics are commonly used to treat acne vulgaris, primarily in patients presenting with moderate to severe facial or truncal disease severity. These agents are most appropriately used in combination with a topical regimen containing benzoyl peroxide and a topical retinoid. The most common oral antibiotics for treating acne vulgaris are the tetracycline derivatives, although macrolide agents such as erythromycin have also been used extensively. Over the past 4 decades, as the sensitivity of Propionibacterium acnes to several oral and topical antibiotics has decreased, the efficacy of oral tetracycline and erythromycin has markedly diminished, leading to increased use of doxycycline, minocycline, and other agents, such as trimethoprim/sulfamethoxazole.

Community-acquired methicillin-resistant Staphylococcus aureus (CA-MRSA) continues to make headlines because of large outbreaks in daycare centers and among members of athletic teams. CA-MRSA infections in children commonly lead to hospitalization. Life-threatening infections, such as necrotizing pneumonitis and brain abscess, can occur. The organism has crossed into hospitals and is now a common cause of hospital-acquired sepsis. Multidrug-resistant strains of MRSA are emerging in Asia, with the resistance based on either a novel gene cassette or a transmissible plasmid. The routine use of antibiotics in livestock seems to be contributing to the emergence of resistant organisms, and some of these have already produced human infection. Fortunately, most cutaneous CA-MRSA infections present as abscesses or furunculosis, and these manifestations generally respond to drainage. The recurrence and attack rates of close contacts are high and relate to persistent colonization.

Sexually transmissible diseases (STDs) remain a major health issue worldwide, with approximately 300 million new cases annually. STDs caused by bacteria can be treated with antibiotics, although the susceptibility pattern of many etiologic microbes has changed over the past few decades. Syphilis remains best managed with single-dose benzathine penicillin G. Other single-dose antibiotic regimens for lues are either associated with clinical failure or of uncertain dosage. However, single-dose azithromycin and ceftriaxone are suitable for chancroid. Lymphogranuloma venereum, reemergent as a cause of proctitis, is treated with prolonged courses of doxycycline or minocycline. Trimethoprim-sulfamethoxazole has replaced tetracycline derivatives as preferred treatment for donovanosis in many regions. Parenteral cephalosporins, such as ceftriaxone, cefotaxime, and ceftizoxime, are initial interventions for disseminated gonococcemia. Pending culture results, genital bite wounds (often consisting of deep, painful ulcerations) should be treated with high-dose amoxicillin-clavulanic acid.

Atypical mycobacterial infections have been a cause of steadily growing infections over the past decades, especially in immunocompromised patients. They are classified by their ability to produce pigment, growth rate, and optimal temperature. *Mycobacterium marinum*, *M kansasii*, and *M avium-intracellulare* are examples of slow-growing mycobacteria. *M fortuitum*, *M chelonei*, and *M abscessus* are examples of rapidly growing mycobacteria. Atypical mycobacteria are ubiquitous in the environment. No specific treatment guidelines exist but a multidrug regimen combined with surgical modalities is often used for therapy.

Dermatologists can decrease unnecessary use of antimicrobial agents by avoiding them in situations wherein good evidence indicates that they are ineffective. Controlled trials indicate that antimicrobial agents are unhelpful in treating cutaneous abscesses, inflamed epidermal cysts, uninfected atopic eczema, and cutaneous ulcers caused by venous insufficiency or diabetes in the absence of significant contiguous soft-tissue inflammation. Prophylactic antibiotics are rarely appropriate for routine dermatologic surgery and are not indicated for patients who have prosthetic joints or vascular grafts. They are recommended only for a small group of patients who have abnormal cardiac valves, and then only with surgery involving clearly infected skin or soft-tissue. Topical antibiotics are no better than white petrolatum in covering sutured wounds, and with moist occlusive dressings, no ointment is necessary.

One fascinating element of medical dermatology is the diversity of available therapeutic agents, and dermatologists are well versed in applying the mechanism of action of a drug to modify a disease process. Oral antibiotics are the ideal example of pharmacologic agents that are effective against inflammatory processes and have obvious roles in infectious diseases.

Oral antibiotics are commonly prescribed by dermatologists in clinical practice. When prescribing an oral antibiotic, as with other systemic medications, it is important to consider potential interactions with other drugs, including over-the-counter medications. The most common drug interaction mechanisms that may lead to clinically significant sequelae are inhibition of GI drug absorption and alterations in drug metabolism. Tetracycline and quinolones undergo chelation interactions with many metal ions found in antacids and mineral supplements. Some macrolides, such as erythromycin, inhibit the hepatic metabolism of many other drugs, increasing the risk for toxicity. Rifampin increases the metabolism of many other drugs, thus predisposing to treatment failure. Drug interactions can only be averted if their potential is understood and recognized in advance.

Dermatologic Clinics

RELATED INTEREST

Advances in Dermatology (Volume 24)
William D. James, MD, *Editor-in-Chief*

THE CLINICS ARE NOW AVAILABLE ONLINE!

Access your subscription at:
www.theclinics.com

Preface

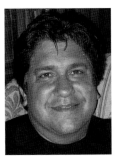

James Q. Del Rosso, DO, FAOCD
Guest Editor

I was honored when Dr. Bruce Thiers invited me to serve as guest editor for this issue of *Dermatologic Clinics*, which is entitled "Antibiotic Use in Dermatology." After forming the Scientific Panel on Antibiotic Use in Dermatology (SPAUD) in 2006, I have continued to remain active academically in this subject area by continuing the SPAUD Project and by participating in other related educational initiatives and publications. I feel it is very important for our specialty to remain vigilant regarding changes in antibiotic susceptibility patterns, emerging pathogens, uses for antibiotics that are unrelated to infectious diseases, and clinical scenarios where it is actually unnecessary to prescribe antibiotic therapy. Importantly, we must continually reconsider how we can optimally utilize antibiotics in order to take maximum advantage of their therapeutic benefits and to reduce the potential for antibiotic resistance.

In this issue of *Dermatologic Clinics*, I have asked several of my colleagues who have a strong interest in antibiotic use in dermatology to contribute clinically pertinent articles. The authors are predominantly "seasoned veterans" in their subject areas. However, I have also called upon a few "rookies" to serve on the team of authors, including Dr. Sanjay Bhambri, chief resident at our dermatology program at Valley Hospital Medical Center in Las Vegas, Nevada. Topics for this issue were selected to bring the reader up to date on a variety of relevant subjects, including acne vulgaris, community-acquired methicillin-resistant Staphylococcus aureus (CA-MRSA)

infection, sexually transmitted diseases, atypical mycobacterial infections, issues related to the use of topical and oral antibiotics, and a review of when antibiotics are unnecessary.

A major "wake-up call" regarding emerging pathogens and antibiotic resistance trends that has essentially rung loudly in every dermatology office across the United States is CA-MRSA. This entity alone has raised significant awareness among dermatologists about how we prescribe antibiotic therapy. In this issue, Dr. Dirk Elston discusses the topic of CA-MRSA and the handling of local outbreaks.

I want to thank all of the contributors to this issue of *Dermatologic Clinics*. Writing quality articles takes a lot of time and is a "labor of love". The efforts of all of the authors are much appreciated. Additionally, all of the publication staff deserve a much appreciated "thank you". Last but not least, my wife Karyn remains continuously supportive of my academic endeavors and is a very inspirational guiding light. Now, please enjoy "Antibiotic Use in Dermatology." All of us who are involved in this issue are hopeful that it will help clinicians provide improved therapy for their patients.

James Q. Del Rosso, DO, FAOCD
Valley Hospital Medical Center
620 Shadow Lane
Las Vegas, NV 89106, USA

E-mail address:
jqdelrosso@yahoo.com

Dermatol Clin 27 (2009) ix
doi:10.1016/j.det.2008.09.001
0733-8635/08/$ – see front matter

Clinical Considerations in the Treatment of Acne Vulgaris and Other Inflammatory Skin Disorders: a Status Report

James J. Leyden, MD[a], James Q. Del Rosso, DO, FAOCD[b],*,
Guy F. Webster, MD, PhD[c]

KEYWORDS

- Antibiotics • Acne vulgaris • Antibiotic resistance
- Anti-inflammatory activity

Propionibacterium acnes is an anaerobic bacterium that plays an important role in the pathogenesis of acne. Certain antibiotics that can inhibit *P acnes* colonization have also demonstrated anti-inflammatory activities in the treatment of acne, rosacea, and other noninfectious diseases. Decreased sensitivity of *P acnes* to antibiotics, such as erythromycin and tetracycline, has developed and may be associated with therapeutic failure. Benzoyl peroxide (BPO) is a non-antibiotic antibacterial agent that is highly effective against *P acnes* and for which no resistance against it has been detected to date. Retinoids are important components in combination therapy for acne, including use with antibiotics, and can serve as an alternative to these agents in maintenance therapy. By increasing our understanding of the multifaceted actions of antibiotics and the known clinical implications of antibiotic resistance, physicians can improve their decision making in prescribing these agents.

Acne vulgaris can be managed with topical or systemic agents, including topical monotherapy, topical combination therapy, or a topical agent combined with systemic drug therapy. Topical treatments include comedolytic agents such as retinoids (ie, adapalene, tazarotene, and tretinoin) and salicylic acid; bactericidal agents such as BPO; and antibiotics such as clindamycin and erythromycin. When a patient is unresponsive to one or a combination of the above treatments, oral antibiotics can be added to the treatment regimen. For severe or recalcitrant acne, other systemic treatments, such as oral isotretinoin and hormonal therapy in women, may be needed.

P acnes is a resident of the normal microflora that can be present in abnormally high numbers in sebaceous follicles of patients with acne and has been implicated in the development of inflammatory acne.[1] A primary mode of action of antibiotic treatment in acne is to decrease the presence of *P acnes* in the skin; however, antibiotics also demonstrate inhibitory effects on the production of *P acnes*–associated inflammatory mediators, and antibiotics likely affect acne by means other than direct antibacterial effects.

Each year, 5 million prescriptions for oral antibiotics and 1.4 million prescriptions for isotretinoin are dispensed for the treatment of acne.[2] Although antibiotic therapy has been used for more than 40 years to treat acne, changes in *P acnes* antibiotic sensitivity did not become an issue until the

[a] University of Pennsylvania, Philadelphia, PA 19104, USA
[b] Valley Hospital Medical Center, 620 Shadow Lane, Las Vegas, NV 89106, USA
[c] Jefferson Medical College, Philadelphia, PA 19107, USA
* Corresponding author. 880 Seven Hills Drive, Suite 260, Henderson, NV 89052.
E-mail address: jqdelrosso@yahoo.com (J.Q. Del Rosso).

Dermatol Clin 27 (2009) 1–15
doi:10.1016/j.det.2008.07.008

1970s.[3] Since then, the prevalence of resistant organisms has increased globally.[4] As a result, clinicians have begun to reevaluate therapeutic approaches with the goal of limiting the development of antibiotic-resistant organisms. This article reviews the anti-inflammatory and nonantimicrobial effects of antibiotics in acne and other diseases and examines issues relating to the emergence of decreased bacterial sensitivity to antibiotics (ie, resistance) and how these issues relate to clinical practice.

MICROBIOLOGY OF *PROPIONIBACTERIUM ACNES*

Human skin is colonized by locally dense or sparse populations of nonpathogenic microorganisms, including coagulase-negative staphylococci and aerobic diphtheroid rods on the skin's surface, and propionibacteria and *Malassezia* yeasts in the infundibulum of the sebaceous follicle. The density and distribution of skin flora vary according to age and environmental factors such as sebum secretion, occlusion, temperature, and humidity.[5] *P acnes* is a facultative anaerobic bacterium that plays an important role in the pathogenesis of acne, which is a complex event arising from the interplay of three pathogenic factors: sebum production, abnormal desquamation of corneocytes in sebaceous follicles, and overgrowth within the pilosebaceous unit by Gram-positive anaerobic *P acnes*. *P acnes* flourishes in the environment created by sebum and follicular cells and produces chemotactic factors and proinflammatory mediators that may lead to inflammation.[6]

Topical application or systemic administration of certain antibiotic agents have demonstrated efficacy in the treatment of acne, the basis of which is to decrease the presence of *P acnes* on the skin and within pilosebaceous follicles. However, the successful treatment of acne also has been attributed to the inhibitory effects of some antibiotics on *P acnes*–associated inflammatory mediators. The anti-inflammatory effects of antibiotics in acne and other diseases are important to consider, both in terms of optimizing treatment effect and in decision making regarding the prescription of these agents in light of antibiotic resistance issues.

The Centers for Disease Control and Prevention established guidelines for the prevention and control of antimicrobial resistance based on the premise that antimicrobial drug use exerts selective pressure favoring resistance and the judicious use of these agents is essential to maximize the life of existing drugs while new drugs are being developed.[7] The recommendations stress the importance of avoiding prescribing antibiotics for viral infections and simple coughs and colds, for which these agents have no effect. However, they make no recommendations for proper prescribing of these agents in inflammatory diseases, where it is primarily the anti-inflammatory actions of these drugs—and not their antimicrobial effects—that contribute to their therapeutic activity. We provide an overview of the anti-inflammatory activities of some antibiotic agents and their potential for use in various dermatologic and nondermatologic diseases.

ANTIBIOTIC USE IN INFLAMMATORY DISEASE

Antibiotics have anti-inflammatory activities, as well as antimicrobial effects, in diseases with or without bacterial etiology. In fact, the idea that certain drugs have multiple effects in the disease process is not new. A well-known example is chloroquine, which initially was used to treat malaria but now is used to treat rheumatoid arthritis, systemic or discoid lupus erythematosus, and other connective tissue disorders.

Commonly prescribed oral antibiotics for acne are tetracyclines; macrolides such as erythromycin; and trimethoprim, with or without sulfamethoxazole. Some of these agents, as well as dapsone, have demonstrated efficacy in various diseases without bacterial etiology.[8–10]

Trimethoprim-Sulfamethoxazole

Trimethoprim-sulfamethoxazole (TMP-SMZ) is an effective treatment in mild Wegener's granulomatous vasculitis,[11] in which case it seems that TMP-SMZ is acting as an anti-inflammatory agent.[10] Furthermore, culture samples for TMP-SMZ–sensitive organisms have been taken in the granuloma of patients but none have been found.[12] Webster[12] and Leyden[13] have shown in unpublished studies that TMP-SMZ is beneficial in the treatment of sterile scalp pustulosis and acne, respectively.

Dapsone

Although structurally distinct from the sulfonamides, dapsone is a sulfone antibiotic agent that inhibits the bacterial synthesis of dihydrofolic acid similar to sulfonamides. The anti-inflammatory effects of dapsone have been recognized for many years, mostly because of its dramatic efficacy in dermatitis herpetiformis[14] which is an immune-mediated disease.[12] Dapsone therapy results in rapid resolution of symptoms, but withdrawal causes a rapid recurrence of the disease. These kinetics suggest that the drug may be functioning as a reversible inhibitor of one or more inflammatory systems.[15] It has been proposed that the anti-inflammatory properties of dapsone in humans are mostly attributed to modulation of polymorphonuclear leukocyte function, such as decreases in myeloperoxidase activity,[10] inhibition of the generation or release of 5-lipoxygenase products,[16] decreases in polymorphonuclear leukocyte adherence,[17] and decreases in α_1-antitrypsin inactivation;[18] each of which are unrelated to the antibiotic action of dapsone.

The sulfonamides and dapsone have demonstrated varying degrees of response against a number of noninfectious inflammatory and bullous diseases (**Box 1**), including pyoderma gangrenosum, linear immunoglobulin A dermatosis, cicatricial pemphigoid, atopic dermatitis, and acne.[10,12,14,15] However, dapsone is not an FDA-approved therapy in all of these diseases. Dapsone use is associated with dose-dependent adverse hematologic reactions such as methemoglobinemia, hemolysis, and anemia, even with the low daily dose of 100 mg used in the treatment of leprosy and dermatologic conditions. Severe idiosyncratic reactions include agranulocytosis and dapsone hypersensitivity syndrome, which is defined by the clinical triad of fever, rash, and internal organ involvement, most commonly the liver and hematologic system. Although dapsone hypersensitivity syndrome occurs in a relatively small proportion of patients, it is associated with considerable morbidity and mortality.[14] Dapsone, however, has resurfaced in topical form as a potential therapeutic agent in acne. Furthermore, clinical experience suggests that problems arising from oral dapsone use, such as neuropathy and bone marrow failure, may be more common in older patients.[12]

There are three types of tetracyclines available: tetracycline natural products, tetracycline semisynthetic compounds, and chemically modified tetracyclines. Although their role in inflammation remains to be defined completely, both laboratory and clinical studies have investigated the anti-inflammatory properties of these agents. **Table 1** summarizes the inhibitory effects of tetracyclines on inflammation.[19]

Importantly, tetracyclines inhibit nitric oxide, which modulates blood flow and white blood cell function in wound healing and inflammation. Nitric oxide participates in inflammatory and autoimmune-mediated tissue destruction, and increased levels of nitric oxide, are found in patients with autoimmune diseases, including rheumatoid arthritis, systemic lupus erythematosus, ulcerative colitis, and Crohn's disease. It also has been demonstrated that several inflammatory symptoms, such as erythema and vascular leakiness, can be reversed by nitric oxide synthetase inhibitors. Tetracyclines have the ability to decrease inflammatory bone and cartilage destruction,[20] and doxycycline and minocycline have demonstrated benefit in experimental cardiovascular accident.[21] A more comprehensive list of therapeutic uses of tetracyclines is provided in **Box 2**. Importantly, anti-inflammatory dose doxycycline is approved by the US Food and Drug Administration for the treatment of inflammatory lesions (papules and pustules) of rosacea in adults. One study has shown that an anti-inflammatory dose of doxycycline is efficacious in mild to moderate acne without having any effect on microorganisms. However, the time required to observe clinical benefit may be longer than when using doses that achieve an antibiotic effect.[12,22]

Box 1
Reported beneficial effects of dapsone and sulfonamides in inflammatory diseases

Sulfonamides and dapsone (sulfapyridine, sulfasalazine)

- Rheumatoid arthritis
- Dermatitis herpetiformis
- Pyoderma gangrenosum
- Weber-Christian panniculitis
- Cystic acne
- Leprosy

Dapsone

- Relapsing polychondritis
- Lupus-associated urticaria
- Erythema elevatum diutinum
- Pustular psoriasis
- Allergic vasculitis
- Herpes gestationis
- Linear immunoglobulin A dermatosis
- Cicatricial pemphigoid
- Atopic dermatitis

Trimethoprim-sulfamethoxazole

- Wegener granulomatosis

Sulfasalazine

- Ankylosing spondylitis
- Reiter's syndrome
- Inflammatory bowel disease

Adapted from Roberts DE, Curd JG. Arthritis Rheum 1990;33:1590–3; with permission.

Table 1
Inhibitory effects of tetracyclines on inflammation

Drug	Inhibitory Effects on Inflammation
TCN, DCN	Inhibition of mitogen-induced human lymphocytic proliferation by blockage of blast transformation
TCN	Suppression of neutrophilic migration and chemotaxis
MCN	Inhibition of transmigration of T lymphocytes and production of MMP-9 in a murine model of autoimmune encephalitis
TCN	Inhibition of inflammatory response following application of potassium iodide
MCN	Inhibition of T-lymphocyte activation, with resultant inhibition of T-cell proliferation
MCN, DCN	Inhibition of phospholipase A_2
MCN	Up-regulation of anti-inflammatory cytokine IL-10 in synovial explants
MCN, DCN, CMT	Inhibition of the expression of nitric oxide synthetase
DCN, CMT-3	Accelerated degradation of nitric oxide synthetase

Abbreviations: CMT, chemically modified tetracycline; DCN, doxycycline; IL-10, interleukin 10; MCN, minocycline; MMP, matrix metalloproteinase; TCN, tetracycline.
From Sapadin AN, Fleischmajer R. Tetracyclines: nonantibiotic properties and their clinical implications. J Am Acad Dermatol 2006;54:258–65; with permission.

The efficacy of oral agents such as tetracyclines in rosacea probably is more related to anti-inflammatory effects than antibiotic activity. Anti-inflammatory effects of oral tetracyclines, especially doxycycline and minocycline, also are believed to contribute to the improvement of acne. Tetracyclines and their analogs inhibit some matrix metalloproteinases (MMPs), which are zinc-dependent endopeptidases that play an important role in the remodeling of connective tissue and are involved in embryogenesis, wound healing, rheumatoid arthritis, and tumor invasion and metastasis.[19,23] There are MMPs that break down fibrillar collagens—that is, collagenases (MMP-1, MMP-8, MMP-13)—and MMPs that affect basement membrane collagen, known as gelatinases (MMP-2, MMP-9). Tetracycline and its analogs can inhibit both collagenases and gelatinases.[19] The inhibition of MMPs by tetracyclines has demonstrated promise in various inflammatory diseases, including embolic disease and ocular rosacea[24,25] and has been shown to suppress periodontal disease without affecting the bacterial flora of the mouth.[26–28] The anti-inflammatory effects of tetracyclines are believed to be of benefit in the treatment of acne and rosacea.

Chemically modified tetracyclines result from modifications of the tetracycline structure, which eliminate antibiotic activity but retain the anti-inflammatory properties, making them effective in treating diseases that involve inflammation or destruction of the body's connective tissues.

Chemically modified tetracyclines have been shown to inhibit tissue-destructive enzymes such as elastase and MMPs (MMP-1, MMP-2, MMP-9, MMP-13) in numerous cell lines, tissues, and in vivo models, as well as the expression of inducible nitric oxide synthetase and the production of nitric oxide. In preclinical models, the chemically modified tetracycline incyclinide was found to prevent acute lung injury, the development of osteoarthritis, the dilation and subsequent development of abdominal aortic aneurysm, and the growth and spread of cancer.[29]

Long-term use of tetracycline antibiotics is often safer than other anti-inflammatory drugs, especially systemic immunosuppressive drugs. Because of their anti-inflammatory activities, these agents are sensible choices for the treatment of chronic noninfectious diseases such as low-grade vasculitis,[12] sarcoidosis,[8] rheumatoid arthritis;[30] and bullous diseases such as bullous pemphigoid[31] and Hailey-Hailey disease.[32]

ANTI-INFLAMMATORY EFFECTS OF ANTIBIOTICS IN ACNE

Topical and oral administration of certain antibiotics have demonstrated efficacy in the treatment of acne, the success of which can be attributed in part to the reduction of the overgrowth of P acnes. However, some antibiotics exert anti-inflammatory effects that also are important in the treatment of this disorder. Although P acnes is the predominant microorganism in the pilosebaceous follicle, this

Box 2
Therapeutic uses of tetracyclines in dermatologic and nondermatologic diseases

Dermatologic diseases

    Acne

    Rosacea

    Bullous dermatoses

    Sarcoidosis

    Kaposi sarcoma

    Pyoderma gangrenosum

    Hidradenitis suppurativa

    Sweet syndrome

    α_1-Antitrypsin deficiency panniculitis

    Pityriasis lichenoides chronica

Nondermatologic diseases

    Rheumatoid arthritis

    Scleroderma

    Cancer

    Cardiovascular diseases

    Abdominal aortic aneurysm

    Acute myocardial infarction

    Periodontitis

From Sapadin AN, Fleischmajer R. Tetracyclines: non-antibiotic properties and their clinical implications. J Am Acad Dermatol 2006;54:258–65; with permission.

organism usually is not pathogenic, which is evident from the lack of correlation between the number of bacteria and the severity and type of acne.[33] However, the inflammatory component in acne appears to be produced by the host response to *P acnes* and its proinflammatory mediators. The anti-inflammatory effects of tetracyclines when used to treat acne appear to be related to decreases in neutrophil chemotaxis[1,34] and the production of chemotactic factors, proinflammatory cytokines,[35,36] and lipase,[37] as well as the down-regulation of several MMP enzymes.[27,28]

MINIMUM INHIBITORY CONCENTRATION

The basic quantitative measure of the in vitro activity of antibiotics is the minimum inhibitory concentration (MIC), which is the lowest concentration of the antibiotic that results in inhibition of visible growth of the organism. However, the MIC of any antibiotic against *P acnes* only partially reflects

potential anti-acne efficacy. MICs are derived from aqueous systems. An important determinant of the efficacy of an antibiotic is the drug's ability to penetrate the lipophilic environment of the sebaceous follicle. *P acnes* is susceptible to a wide range of antibiotics, but over the years, it has become clear that not all antibiotics are equally effective in penetrating the lipid-filled microcomedone and reducing the number of *P acnes* in the skin. However, drugs that are more lipophilic (eg, doxycycline, minocycline) are better able to penetrate the sebaceous follicle and, as a result, are more efficient in reducing *P acnes*.[38]

An example of the lack of correlation between the MIC of a drug and its clinical efficacy is BPO. It is well known that BPO is effective in reducing *P acnes* counts, but BPO is a highly lipophilic molecule with a high MIC (150 µg/mL) that does not perform well in an aqueous system. Consequently, its MIC is not indicative of the efficacy of this agent against *P acnes*.[13] Another problem in interpreting MICs is that the follicular concentration of antibiotics is unknown. Although we do not have a better way to predict the clinical efficacy of a particular agent other than MIC, it is possible that many potentially useful acne drugs have been excluded erroneously over the years because of their high MICs determined in aqueous systems.

Some antibiotics are capable of reducing the inflammatory capacity of *P acnes* without inhibiting the growth of the organism. This is accomplished by using sub-MICs of an antibiotic, which means dosing below the established drug level or MIC that is necessary to achieve antibiotic effect. Skidmore and colleagues[22] showed that a sub-antimicrobial dose of doxycycline demonstrated significant reductions in the number of inflammatory and noninflammatory lesions (P<.01) in subjects with moderate facial acne. In addition to the reductions in lesion counts, these investigators found that treatment did not demonstrate any detectable effect on skin flora, colonization of the skin by opportunistic pathogens, or any increase in the number or severity of resistant organisms.[22]

Sub-MICs of other antibiotics also have demonstrated anti-inflammatory effects. Webster and colleagues[37] demonstrated inhibition of lipase production in *P acnes* by sub-MICs of tetracycline and erythromycin. In another study by Webster and colleagues,[35] sub-MIC concentrations of tetracycline, erythromycin, ampicillin, and minocycline were able to reduce the inflammatory capacity of *P acnes* by suppressing polymorphonuclear leukocyte chemotactic factor production in the organism. Although the clinical significance of these results remains to be fully elucidated, it is possible that these antibiotics could serve as adjunctive therapy in atopic dermatitis, periodontitis, and other diseases for which increasing severity is proportional to increases in bacterial colonization of affected areas. The ability of an antibiotic to reduce the inflammatory capacity of the organism could enhance clinical improvement.[35]

ANTIBIOTICS IN CHRONIC INFLAMMATORY DISEASE

It still is unclear how antibiotics affect the chronic inflammatory response, which may be an important consideration in the treatment of severe acne. In particular, the granulomatous response is poorly understood. It is possible to produce granulomas in animal models by the injection of particulate stimuli. These particles induce granulomalike formations in vitro. This phenomenon has been studied by Webster and colleagues.[39] They assessed the ability of commonly used antibiotics in an in vitro model of granuloma formation. They induced formation of granulomas by incubating peripheral blood mononuclear cells with dextran beads either in or without the presence of various antibiotics. Results showed that the antibiotics commonly used in acne (eg, tetracycline, doxycycline, minocycline) demonstrated reasonable suppression of granuloma formation, with doxycycline and minocycline almost being equivalent. Furthermore, the results showed that these drugs were inactive in the granuloma model had no effect on protein kinase C activity. The tetracyclines and ciprofloxacin all caused dose-dependent inhibition of protein kinase C activity in the same order of relative potency as was found for the inhibition of granuloma formation (**Table 2**). These results are especially interesting because the antigranuloma activity of each drug corresponds to the clinical efficacy of these agents in the treatment of severe acne and inflammatory

rosacea. That is, doxycycline and minocycline are most efficacious in these disorders; tetracycline and ciprofloxacin are weakly efficacious; and erythromycin, ampicillin, and the cephalosporins, which are not as effective in acne vulgaris, do not inhibit protein kinase C.[39]

The clinical application of these observations is that antibiotics often are safer than other antiinflammatory drugs, such as corticosteroids and cytotoxic agents, for long-term treatment of inflammatory diseases; and they are sensible choices for the treatment of diseases such as low-grade vasculitis, sarcoid ulcers, and bullous pemphigoid. Furthermore, the positive effects of antibiotics, primarily minocycline, in rheumatoid arthritis have been demonstrated.[30] Antibiotics may be a less toxic treatment alternative and a potential tool to reduce corticosteroid use in some chronic inflammatory diseases, which mandates the further study of their anti-inflammatory activity and potential for disease modification.

PROPIONIBACTERIUM ACNES RESISTANCE

It is clear that in the past 20 years, the sensitivity of P acnes to macrolides (erythromycin), clindamycin, and tetracyclines has substantially changed. In many cases, acne vulgaris may respond to antibiotic therapy slowly, or it may require prolonged maintenance therapy. These factors, combined with the fact that topical and oral antibiotics have been widely prescribed for more than 40 years, has resulted in selection pressure whereby antibiotics kill susceptible bacteria that allow antibiotic-resistant bacteria to survive, multiply, and proliferate over time. Although some bacteria are inherently resistant to certain types of antibiotics, bacteria also may become resistant by a genetic mutation or by acquiring resistance transferred from another organism.

Table 2 Inhibition of protein kinase C by antibiotics	
Antibiotic	Inhibition (%)
Tetracycline	79
Doxycycline	99
Minocycline	83
Ciprofloxacin	50
Erythromycin, ampicillin, cephalosporin, clindamycin	<5

Adapted from Webster GF, Toso SM, Hegemann L. Inhibition of a model of in vitro granuloma formation by tetracyclines and ciprofloxacin. involvement of protein kinase C. Arch Dermatol 1994;130:748–52; with permission.

Propionibacterium acnes Resistance at the Molecular Level

Antibiotic resistance can develop when bacteria acquire mobile genetic elements such as plasmids that can be transferred between strains of species and, less often, between species.[40] In the case of erythromycin and tetracyclines, these plasmids and transposons, or "jumping genes," alternate targets of antibiotics or encode permeases that pump antibiotics back out of the host cell. In the case of clinically relevant strains of resistant P acnes, mobile elements have not been found. Instead, point mutations in the genes encoding the 23S ribosomal RNA (rRNA; erythromycin) and the 16S rRNA (tetracycline) have been identified. Table 3 lists the phenotypes of erythromycin-resistant and tetracycline-resistant P acnes. Three mutations have been described for erythromycin; for tetracycline, there is one mutation in the 16S segment.[40]

Mutations in the 23S rRNA component of Escherichia coli–equivalent nucleotide bases lead to varying degrees of resistance to erythromycin and clindamycin. For example, mutations at E coli–equivalent base 2057 create low levels of resistance to erythromycin and no resistance to clindamycin. In contrast, mutations at E coli–equivalent base 2058 create high levels of resistance to erythromycin and varying degrees of resistance to both clindamycin and other macrolides, whereas mutations at E coli–equivalent base 2059 create high levels of resistance to erythromycin and variable resistance to clindamycin.[40] As a result of these mutations, most strains of P acnes that are resistant to erythromycin may be cross-resistant to clindamycin.[41] In one study,

18 (64%) subjects who previously had been treated with oral erythromycin had an increase in erythromycin-resistant propionibacteria when treated with topical clindamycin compared with 5 (20%) subjects with no prior treatment.[42] However, further clarification on how resistance develops is needed. There are likely other mutations because some insensitive strains do not have these mutations.[4]

Whether a bacteria-acquired resistance gene occurs by mutation or by genetic exchange with other bacteria, the organism has the ability to resist one or more antibiotics. Because bacteria can accumulate multiple resistance traits over time, they can become resistant to many different types of antibiotics. However, these resistance traits can be reversed. If the selection pressure exerted by the presence of an antibiotic is removed, the bacterial population potentially could revert to a responsive population of bacteria.

Propionibacterium acnes Resistance at the Global Level

It generally is recognized that P acnes antibiotic sensitivity patterns are changing worldwide. During the past 20 years, there has been a gradual increase in P acnes resistance to various antibiotics. Before that time, therapeutic failure caused by antibiotic-resistant P acnes was uncommon. In 1976, Leyden[43] did not find antibiotic-resistant propionibacteria on the skin of more than 1000 subjects with acne. Later studies reported isolated antibiotic-resistant P acnes in two treatment groups that used either topical erythromycin 1% or topical clindamycin, and the incidence has been steadily increasing since then.[44]

Table 3
Propionibacterium acnes antibiotic resistance

Erythromycin	Mutations in the Genes Encoding 23S rRNA
Group 1	A→G transition at Escherichia coli equivalent base 2058 Highly resistant to erythromycin Variable to other macrolides and clindamycin
Group 2	G→A transition at E coli equivalent base 2057 Low level of erythromycin resistance
Group 3	A→G transition at equivalent base 2059 Highly resistant to erythromycin and all macrolides Elevated but variable resistance to clindamycin
Tetracycline	Mutation in the Gene Encoding 16S rRNA G→C transition at E coli equivalent base 1058 Variable resistance to tetracycline, doxycycline, and minocycline

Abbreviation: rRNA, ribosomal RNA.
From Eady EA, Gloor M, Leyden JJ. Propionibacterium acnes resistance: a worldwide problem. Dermatology 2003;206:54–6; with permission.

Additional studies show that there is *P acnes* resistance in other parts of the world. In a Singapore study, Tan and colleagues[45] found that long-term antibiotic use (>18 weeks) was associated with increased *P acnes* resistance to erythromycin. In France, Dreno and colleagues[46] found that the prevalence of bacterial resistance to erythromycin was 95% for *Staphylococcus epidermidis* strains and 52% for *P acnes* strains. These investigators found that resistant strains were more frequent in subjects with predominantly inflammatory lesions, and even subjects with no previous erythromycin use had resistant strains for *P acnes* (42%).

In a study by Ross and colleagues,[4] the phenotypes and genotypes of 73 antibiotic-resistant strains of *P acnes* obtained from the skin of subjects with acne in the United Kingdom, the United States, France, Germany, Australia, and Japan were compared. Results showed that 23S and 16S mutations that confer antibiotic resistance in *P acnes* are distributed throughout much of the world. In addition, these investigators isolated resistant strains for which mutations could not be identified, which suggests that resistance mechanisms have evolved that have yet to be characterized.

In a more recent study by Ross and colleagues[47] investigators sought to determine the prevalence of skin colonization by antibiotic-resistant propionibacteria among 664 subjects with acne and their contacts in the United Kingdom, Spain, Italy, Greece, Sweden, and Hungary. Results showed the prevalence of carriage of isolates resistant to at least one antibiotic ranged from 51% in Hungary to 94% in Spain. Combined resistance to erythromycin and clindamycin was more common (highest prevalence [Spain], 91%) than resistance to tetracyclines (highest prevalence [United Kingdom], 26.4%), with no isolates resistant to tetracycline detected in Italy or Hungary. Furthermore, the prevalence of resistant propionibacteria on the skin of untreated contacts of the subjects varied from 41% in Hungary to 86% in Spain. The fact that resistant strains can be found in a large percentage of patients is finding more and more support in the literature.[40,47]

PROBLEMS IDENTIFYING THE CLINICAL SIGNIFICANCE OF *PROPIONIBACTERIUM ACNES* RESISTANCE

Although it is clear that less-sensitive strains are emerging progressively worldwide, there are variations in sensitivity patterns among different antibiotics and the clinical significance of *P acnes* resistance has yet to be fully explained. The traditional approach to assessing the clinical significance of less-sensitive strains is to compare the MIC of the antibiotic with the achievable concentration in the body compartment in which the organism is proliferating. However, such break points have not been established because the follicular concentration of antibiotics has yet to be quantified. As discussed, there are limitations in interpreting the clinical relevance of MIC because it is an aqueous-based system, which is not an ideal measure in the lipid-rich environment of the organism. As a result, scientists have had to resort to performing difficult clinical outcome studies that assess patients treated with antibiotics to which *P acnes* are insensitive.[42] Nevertheless, there are data supporting that patients with resistant *P acnes* strains may be more prone to having a poor clinical outcome.[40,42,48]

EVIDENCE FOR CLINICAL RELEVANCE OF RESISTANCE

More than 20 years ago, Leyden and colleagues[49] showed that patients with acne with resistant strains had higher counts of *P acnes* and poorer response to therapy compared with patients with sensitive strains. Soon after, Eady and colleagues[42] demonstrated that the use of oral erythromycin or topical clindamycin encouraged the development of resistant propionibacteria and that the emergence of resistant strains is associated with therapeutic failure in erythromycin-treated patients. On the other hand, despite the observation of increased prevalence of erythromycin-resistant *P acnes* strains and potential for cross-resistance with clindamycin, a 12-week pivotal trial evaluating both topical clindamycin foam and aqueous gel formulations in the treatment of acne vulgaris demonstrated a high degree of clinical efficacy, though the prevalence of *P acnes*–resistant strains in the treated populations was not evaluated.[50] Eady and colleagues[40] conducted an extensive literature review of antibiotic-resistant propionibacteria that revealed methodologic weaknesses in prevalence studies and a paucity of evidence on the clinical significance of antibiotic-resistant organisms. However, rather than conclude that the clinical significance of antibiotic-resistant organisms is of little concern, these results highlight how little we still know about the different strains of *P acnes* and how resistance spreads. While we continue to investigate the import of these resistant organisms to treatment outcomes, prudent antibiotic prescribing is warranted. It also is important to consider how available therapies act and complement each other and how these agents can work together to lessen the potential for antibiotic resistance. For example, concomitant use of BPO has been shown to reduce the emergence of erythromycin-resistant and clindamycin-resistant *P acnes* strains.[48,51,52]

COMMONLY USED THERAPIES FOR ACNE

Many topical therapies have been successfully used in the treatment of acne, including formulations of erythromycin, clindamycin, azelaic acid, BPO, and combinations of BPO with erythromycin or clindamycin.[6,53,54] Erythromycin and clindamycin are the most commonly used topical antibiotics for acne.[55] Topical antibiotics such as clindamycin remain an important component of combination treatment for acne vulgaris because of their ability to augment the therapeutic response when used in combination with BPO or a topical retinoid. However, the use of antibiotics as prolonged monotherapy should be avoided for treatment of acne because long-term use is associated with the emergence of resistant bacterial organisms.[56] One study demonstrated the increase in the emergence of resistant *P acnes* strains beginning after 8 weeks of topical antibiotic monotherapy for acne, with the number of resistant strains increasing substantially progressively during the 16-week study.[48]

Concomitant use of BPO with erythromycin or clindamycin is recommended because combination therapy increases efficacy compared with the use of either agent alone, and BPO provides the additional benefits of not being associated with *P acnes* resistance and reducing the emergence of erythromycin-resistant or clindamycin-resistant *P acnes* strains.[51,52,57] **Fig. 1** shows the reduction in *P acnes* with topical therapy and the increased effectiveness of combination therapies in reducing *P acnes*.[38] Although the additive mechanisms of combination therapy are not clear, the concomitant use of BPO with a topical antibiotic, especially clindamycin, is highly effective in reducing the colony counts of cutaneous *P acne*.[54,57,58]

Antibiotic monotherapy, especially for the long-term, is not recommended in the treatment of acne vulgaris. Prolonged topical or oral antibiotic therapy for acne vulgaris is best accompanied by the use of benzoyl peroxide to optimize efficacy and mitigate the emergence of less sensitive *Propionibacterium acnes* strains.

Retinoids

Retinoids are useful agents in the treatment of acne, whether using a topical retinoid as part of a treatment regimen for mild to moderate acne or an oral isotretinoin in the treatment of recalcitrant acne. Topical retinoids can be used alone or in combination with antibiotics or BPO in mild to moderate acne. Topical retinoids also appear to be an option for maintenance therapy in acne because they exhibit anti-inflammatory and anticomedonal activities.[56] Recently, the efficacy of the topical retinoids adapalene and tazarotene was assessed. Thiboutot and colleagues[59] evaluated the maintenance effect of adapalene gel versus vehicle in subjects with severe acne who had been successfully treated with a combination of adapalene gel and doxycycline. Adapalene used as maintenance therapy resulted in significantly higher maintenance rates (75% versus 54%; $P < .001$) and significantly lower noninflammatory ($P = .02$) and inflammatory ($P = .01$) lesion counts.

Similarly, Leyden and colleagues[60] assessed the efficacy of three regimens—topical tazarotene, oral minocycline hydrochloride, or both—as maintenance therapy in moderately severe to severe acne. While a volunteer sample of 189 subjects with moderately severe to severe acne vulgaris were enrolled in the initial 12-week study, 110 subjects entered a maintenance phase of the study for an additional 12 weeks. Ninety subjects completed the maintenance phase and only two

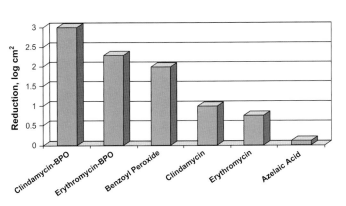

Fig. 1. Reduction of *Propionibacterium acnes* with topical therapy (twice daily treatment for 6 weeks). (*From* Leyden JJ. The evolving role of Propionibacterium acnes in acne. Semin Cutan Med Surg 2001;20:139–43; with permission.)

discontinued because of adverse events. Results showed that each of these regimens was effective in sustaining improvement. After 12 weeks of therapy, the mean reductions in noninflammatory and inflammatory lesion counts from baseline were 60% and 54%, respectively, with tazarotene (n = 36); 52% and 66%, respectively, with minocycline; and 64% and 66%, respectively, with tazarotene plus minocycline (n = 37). The difference in efficacy between the combination of tazarotene alone versus tazarotene and minocycline was not statistically significant.[60]

The fact that a high number of patients who present with a more severe grade of acne can be adequately controlled after a marked degree of improvement has been achieved is strong support for using a topical retinoid during maintenance therapy and underscores the importance of continued adherence to treatment. This approach may help to minimize the duration of long-term antibiotic therapy in some patients. Depending on the individual case, topical maintenance treatment also may include the use of BPO and topical antibiotics.

The combined use of BPO, a topical or oral antibiotic, and a topical retinoid is rational for acne management. Long-term use of a topical retinoid—with or without use of BPO and a topical antibiotic, depending on the individual case—is effective for long-term maintenance treatment in many patients after adequate disease control is achieved. If topical or oral antibiotics are used long-term, the Scientific Panel on Antibiotic Use in Dermatology recommends concomitant use of a BPO-containing formulation to sustain long-term response. Whenever possible, the duration of long-term oral antibiotic therapy for acne or rosacea should be limited as much as is clinically feasible.

Oral Antibiotics

Systemic antibiotics are indicated in cases of moderate to severe acne and for acne resistant to topical therapy alone. Lipophilic antibiotics, especially doxycycline or minocycline, are more effective in reducing the number of P acnes when delivered orally (**Fig. 2**). The therapeutic effects of orally administered antibiotics, such as tetracyclines, include the suppression of P acnes and its anti-inflammatory properties.[54]

Tetracyclines and the macrolide agent erythromycin have been associated with a decrease in neutrophil chemotaxis and the production of chemotactic factors.[35] Doxycycline and minocycline are especially effective during the inflammatory stage of acne.[19,22] Although definitive comparative clinical studies of oral antibiotics used to treat acne vulgaris are limited, the second-generation tetracyclines such as doxycycline and minocycline induce a quicker clinical response than first-generation tetracyclines.[56]

Among the oral antibiotics used to treat acne vulgaris, minocycline exhibits the greatest degree of P acnes reduction, which is likely related to its greater lipophilicity compared with other oral tetracyclines.[61] Interestingly, the use of an extended-release formulation of oral minocycline for the treatment of acne vulgaris based on patient weight has demonstrated that an average daily dose of 1 mg/kg is equal in efficacy to a daily dose of 2 and 3 mg/kg, with the lower dose being associated with a reduced risk of vestibular side effects.[62]

Isotretinoin is a synthetic retinoid and is unique because it can reverse all aspects of acne pathogenesis, including its ability to substantially reduce P acnes–resistant organisms on the skin.[56] Coates and colleagues[63] showed that isotretinoin can effectively reduce the colonization of antibiotic-resistant propionibacteria both on the skin and in the nares in patients with acne. Isotretinoin is indicated for the treatment of severe recalcitrant nodular acne and generally should be reserved for use in patients who have shown inadequate response to other conventional therapies, including one or more systemic antibiotics.

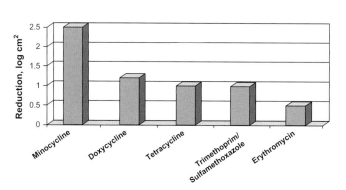

Fig. 2. Reduction in *Propionibacterium acnes* with oral therapy. (*From* Leyden JJ. The evolving role of Propionibacterium acnes in acne. Semin Cutan Med Surg 2001;20:139–43; with permission.)

Although topical and oral antibiotic therapy may impact the microbiologic flora of the skin and nares, data are more limited with topical antibiotic use, especially in regard to clinical significance. Further study is needed in this area to better differentiate implications that may be clinically significant to both individual patients and the general population. Despite the need for additional research in this area, it is clear that the prevalence of resistant organisms is growing steadily.

The presence of less sensitive P acnes organisms may contribute to decreased efficacy of antibiotic treatment in some patients, especially if a high density of less sensitive strains is present. However, oral antibiotics such as doxycycline and minocycline, as well as topical clindamycin, have continued to maintain efficacy in many patients, specifically when used in appropriate combination with other agents, such as benzoyl peroxide and topical retinoids.

There are many ways that the clinician can reduce the potential for P acnes resistance and, at the same time, maximize treatment outcomes. The duration of antibiotic therapy should be limited whenever possible, but if prolonged topical or oral antibiotic therapy is necessary it is best to use the antibiotic in combination with BPO to optimize efficacy and limit the potential for P acnes resistance. Topical retinoids should be used early in the treatment course because they may allow for a shorter course of antibiotics in some patients, especially during the maintenance phase of treatment. In fact, the combination of BPO, a topical or oral antibiotic, and a topical retinoid is a rational treatment approach. The retinoid can be used for long-term maintenance after adequate response has been achieved.

Although clinicians must take steps to minimize the selection pressures on P acnes, this does not mean that the therapeutic efficacy of acne regimens has to be compromised. Antibiotics have important antibacterial and anti-inflammatory effects in acne and other cutaneous diseases, and these agents should continue to be efficacious, provided they are used appropriately.

CURRENT CONTROVERSIES ON LONG-TERM ANTIBIOTIC USE FOR ACNE

Because antibiotics frequently are used in the long-term treatment of acne, patients receiving this therapy serve as a useful natural model to determine if concern about the emergence of resistant organisms and if their negative impact on treatment outcomes in acne extends to other infectious illnesses. Some controversial examples of such ecological mischief include a possible association between erythromycin treatment and an increase of coagulase-negative staphylococci, an increased risk of upper respiratory tract infection (URTI), and the association of long-term antibiotic acne treatment with the oropharyngeal colonization of resistant streptococcal organisms.

Concerns regarding antibiotic use for acne vulgaris are not limited to the development of P acnes resistance. A more recent issue that relates to long-term antibiotic use is the potential for selection pressure or transfer of the resistant genes to potentially pathogenic bacteria, such as certain strains of staphylococci or streptococci. Two studies addressed the effects of topical erythromycin therapy on the ecology of aeobic cutaneous bacterial flora. These studies showed that topical erythromycin use increased erythromycin-resistant coagulase-negative staphylococci on both the treated and distant sites.[64,65] Treating the face with erythromycin increased the prevalence and density of organisms not only on the face but also on the back and anterior nares. Furthermore, Vowels and colleagues[64] found that the prevalence and density of these resistant organisms persisted even after discontinuation of treatment with topical erythromycin and did not return to baseline values until 6 weeks posttreatment. Although the clinical impact of these results is unknown, a point of further study would be to assess if using BPO in combination with erythromycin or clindamycin has any effect on the antibiotic sensitivity patterns of staphylococcal or streptococcal skin organisms.

Another report of possible ecological mischief is the potential for long-term antibiotic treatment for acne to increase a patient's susceptibility for infection. In a retrospective study, Margolis and colleagues[66] examined if the long-term use of antibiotics for acne resulted in the increase of URTI and urinary tract infections (UTI). These investigators identified 118,496 subjects with acne, of which 84,977 (72%) were treated with a topical or oral antibiotic (ie, tetracyclines, erythromycin, clindamycin) and 33,519 (28%) were not treated with a topical or oral antibiotic. Results showed that 15% of all subjects with acne had at least one URTI, and the odds of developing a URTI among subjects receiving antibiotic treatment were 2.15 times greater (95% CI, 2.05–2.23; P<.001) than those who were not receiving antibiotic therapy (**Table 4**). Because of the rarity of UTIs in men, multivariable regression models were not possible for this group. However, multivariable logistic regression for women showed that there was no statistically significant association between antibiotic use and UTI.

Table 4
Association of antibiotic treatment of acne and upper respiratory tract infection

Variable Evaluated	No Antibiotic Used (n = 33,519)	Antibiotic Used (n = 84,977)	P Value
URTI, n (%)	3096 (9.2)	15,185 (18.6)	<.001
UTI, n (%)	1258 (3.8)	3012 (3.5)	.08
Females, n (%)	21,507 (64.2)	44,725 (52.6)	<.001

From Mills O, Thornsberry C, Cardin CW, et al. Bacterial resistance and therapeutic outcome following three months of topical acne therapy with 2% erythromycin gel versus its vehicle. Acta Derm Venereol 2002;82:260–5; with permission.

There are limitations with the methodology of this study that prevent the drawing of definitive conclusions about the effect of antibiotic use and the increased rate of infection. The limitations include the following: (1) the analysis was retrospective, based on diagnosis coding, and there was a failure to assess URTI history in the study population (investigators could not obtain a confirmed diagnosis of bacterial URTI); and (2) the number of subjects treated with topical antibiotics alone was small. Of those subjects who used antibiotics, 6.1% used topical agents alone, 1.3% used oral agents alone, and 92.6% used a combination of topical and oral agents. Definitive conclusions regarding the relationship of topical antibiotic therapy for acne and the risk of URTI cannot be made; further study is needed.

Levy and colleagues[67] sought to estimate the prevalence and resistance patterns of *Staphylococcus aureus* and *Streptococcus pyogenes* in the oropharynx of subjects treated with topical or oral antibiotics for at least 3 months versus subjects not treated with antibiotics for 6 months or more. Of the 105 subjects who participated in this study, 42 subjects were using topical or oral antibiotics and 63 subjects were not using antibiotics. Study results showed that there was a 3-fold greater risk of *S pyogenes* colonization

in the oropharynx in subjects using any antibiotic therapy versus subjects not using antibiotic therapy. However, the prevalence of *S pyogenes* in the nonantibiotic group was higher than expected. Lower percentages of subjects who were positive for *S aureus* were found in groups using any antibiotic, but a higher percentage of subjects who were not using antibiotics had *S aureus* colonization compared with *S pyogenes* colonization (**Table 5**). Finally, 11 of 13 (85%) *S pyogenes* cultures from subjects using antibiotics were resistant to at least one tetracycline antibiotic (ie, tetracycline, doxycycline, minocycline) compared with 1 of 5 (20%) subjects not using antibiotics.

The development of tetracycline-resistant cutaneous flora is a documented consequence of antibiotic therapy for acne, and previous studies also have shown high rates of cross-resistance to other antibiotics such as penicillin, ampicillin, and clindamycin.[63,64] Furthermore, there is evidence that relatives of patients using oral tetracyclines may harbor increased levels of tetracycline-resistant bowel[68] and skin flora.[69] Further study could determine if this increased resistance in close contacts of patients with acne on long-term antibiotic therapy would extend to increased resistance of the oropharyngeal flora.

Table 5
Prevalence of *Streptococcus pyogenes* and *Staphylococcus aureus* in the oropharynx of individuals with acne using antibiotics versus those not using antibiotics

Antibiotic Use	S Pyogenes[a]	P Value	S Aureus[a]	P Value
None	6/63 (10)	Referent	18/62 (29)	Referent
Any	13/39 (33)	.003	9/41 (22)	.42
Oral only	5/18 (28)	.05	4/20 (20)	.43
Topical only	4/10 (40)	.01	2/10 (20)	.55
Both oral and topical	4/11 (36)	.02	3/11 (27)	.91

[a] Number of subjects/potential number of subjects (percentage).

Limitations of the Levy and colleagues[67] study are the number of antibiotic-treated subjects (n = 39) and the small number of subjects treated with a topical antibiotic alone (n = 10) that were available for analysis. Definitive conclusions on the activities of topical versus oral antibiotics in terms of their potential effects on the microbial equilibrium cannot be made from such a relatively small study population. However, because of the potential significance of the findings in this study, a large scale, well-designed, longitudinal trial is warranted to examine the clinical implications of these findings.

Presently, there is limited data. As a result, it would be premature to conclude that patients with acne who are on a long-term antibiotic regimen are more susceptible to infection. However, additional study is warranted to determine if long-term antibiotic therapy, such as what may be used for the treatment of acne and rosacea, increases the development of resistant organisms associated with infections such as URTI and causes an increased incidence of such infections.

SUMMARY

Antibiotics have important antibacterial and anti-inflammatory activities that are useful in treating both infectious and noninfectious cutaneous diseases, including acne and rosacea. The prevention of bacterial resistance in patients with dermatologic disease is an important goal of therapy in patients with disorders such as acne and rosacea, especially because these chronic conditions likely will require a prolonged course of therapy. It has been demonstrated that *P acnes*–resistant organisms may be associated with therapeutic failure in some patients with acne, and the prudent use of antibiotics is necessary to ensure that we can continue to use these drugs to combat disease effectively. Fortunately, there are treatment strategies that can effectively minimize the potential for development of resistant *P acnes* organisms. Antibiotics should be prescribed only for diseases in which they exhibit clinical benefit. Monotherapy with topical and oral antibiotics for acne should be avoided. If long-term therapy is necessary to achieve an adequate therapeutic result, use of BPO with topical or oral antibiotic therapy is recommended. Topical retinoids are an important and effective component of both initial treatment and long-term acne maintenance therapy, and they may be used effectively in combination with BPO and antibiotics to accelerate response. Finally, anti-inflammatory dose doxycycline is an effective treatment option for rosacea that does not have any effect on microorganisms.

REFERENCES

1. Webster GF. Acne vulgaris. BMJ 2002;325:475–9.
2. Stern RS. Medication and medical service utilization for acne 1995–1998. J Am Acad Dermatol 2000;43: 1042–8.
3. Leyden JJ, Marples RR, Mills OH, et al. Gram-negative folliculitis—a complication of antibiotic therapy in acne vulgaris. Br J Dermatol 1973;88: 533–48.
4. Ross JI, Snelling AM, Eady EA, et al. Phenotypic and genotypic characterization of antibiotic-resistant *Propionibacterium acnes* isolated from acne patients attending dermatology clinics in Europe, the USA, Japan and Australia. Br J Dermatol 2001; 144:339–46.
5. Elsner P. Antimicrobials and the skin physiological and pathological flora. Curr Probl Dermatol 2006; 33:35–41.
6. Leyden JJ. Therapy for acne vulgaris. N Engl J Med 1997;336:1156–62.
7. Bell DM, Drotman DP. Confronting antimicrobial resistance: a shared goal of family physicians and the CDC. Am Fam Physician [serial online] 1999; 59:2097–8 2100. Available at: http://www.aafp.org/afp/99041ap/editorials.html Accessed August 21, 2006.
8. Bachelez H, Senet P, Cadranel J, et al. The use of tetracyclines for the treatment of sarcoidosis. Arch Dermatol 2001;137:69–73.
9. Abrutyn E. New uses for old drugs. Infect Dis Clin North Am 1989;3:653–4.
10. Roberts DE, Curd JG. Sulfonamides as anti-inflammatory agents in the treatment of Wegener's granulomatosis. Arthritis Rheum 1990;33:1590–3.
11. Valeriano-Marcet J, Spiera H. Treatment of Wegener's granulomatosis with sulfamethoxazole-trimethoprim. Arch Intern Med 1991;151:1649–52.
12. Webster GF. Anti-inflammatory activity of antibiotics. Presented at the Scientific Panel on Antibiotic Use in Dermatology (SPAUD) Meeting. Las Vegas, NV, April 22–23, 2006.
13. Leyden JJ. Antibiotic therapy in acne and rosacea. Presented at the Scientific Panel on Antibiotic Use in Dermatology (SPAUD) Meeting. Las Vegas, NV, April 22–23, 2006.
14. Wolf R, Matz H, Orion E, et al. Dapsone. Dermatol Online J 2002;8:2.
15. Webster GF, Alexander JC, McArthur WP, et al. Inhibition of chemiluminescence in human neutrophils by dapsone. Br J Dermatol 1984;110:657–63.
16. Wozel G, Lehmann B. Dapsone inhibits the generation of 5-lipoxygenase products in human

polymorphonuclear leukocytes. Skin Pharmacol 1995;8:196–202.

17. Modschiedler K, Weller M, Wörl P, et al. Dapsone and colchicine inhibit adhesion of neutrophilic granulocytes to epidermal sections. Arch Dermatol Res 2000;292:32–6.

18. Ottonello L, Dapino P, Scirocco MC, et al. Sulphonamides as anti-inflammatory agents: old drugs for new therapeutic strategies in neutrophilic inflammation? Clin Sci (Lond) 1995;88:331–6.

19. Sapadin AN, Fleischmajer R. Tetracyclines: nonantibiotic properties and their clinical implications. J Am Acad Dermatol 2006;54:258–65.

20. Amin AR, Attur MG, Thakker GD, et al. A novel mechanism of action of tetracyclines: effects on nitric oxide synthases. Proc Natl Acad Sci U S A 1996;93:14014–9.

21. Yrjänheikki J, Keinänen R, Pellikka M, et al. Tetracyclines inhibit microglial activation and are neuroprotective in global brain ischemia. Proc Natl Acad Sci U S A 1998;95:15769–74.

22. Skidmore R, Kovach R, Walker C, et al. Effects of subantimicrobial-dose doxycycline in the treatment of moderate acne. Arch Dermatol 2003;139:459–64.

23. Stetler-Stevenson WG, Liotta LA, Kleiner DE Jr. Extracellular matrix 6: role of matrix metalloproteinases in tumor invasion and metastasis. FASEB J 1993;7:1434–41.

24. Palei AC, Zaneti RA, Fortuna GM, et al. Hemodynamic benefits of matrix metalloproteinase-9 inhibition by doxycycline during experimental acute pulmonary embolism. Angiology 2005;56:611–7.

25. Sobrin L, Liu Z, Monroy DC, et al. Regulation of MMP-9 activity in human tear fluid and corneal epithelial culture supernatant. Invest Ophthalmol Vis Sci 2000;41:1703–9.

26. Golub LM, Lee HM, Ryan ME, et al. Tetracyclines inhibit connective tissue breakdown by multiple non-antimicrobial mechanisms. Adv Dent Res 1998;12:12–26.

27. Golub LM, Ciancio S, Ramamurthy NS, et al. Low-dose doxycycline therapy: effect on gingival and crevicular fluid collagenase activity in humans. J Periodont Res 1990;25:321–30.

28. Grenier D, Plamondon P, Sorsa T, et al. Inhibition of proteolytic, serpinolytic and progelatinase-b activation activities of peridontopathogens by doxycycline and the non-antimicrobial chemically modified tetracycline derivatives. J Periodontol 2002;73:79–85.

29. Core Technologies. CollaGenex Pharmaceuticals Inc Web site. Available at: http://www.collagenex.com/core.asp. Accessed August 18, 2006.

30. O'Dell JR, Paulsen G, Haire CE, et al. Treatment of early seropositive rheumatoid arthritis with minocycline: four-year followup of a double-blind, placebo-controlled trial. Arthritis Rheum 1999;42:1691–5.

31. Loo WJ, Kirtschig G, Wojnarowska F. Minocycline as a therapeutic option in bullous pemphigoid. Clin Dermatol 2001;26:376–9.

32. Helm TN, Lee TC. Familial benign pemphigus (Hailey-Hailey disease) [serial online]. Updated March 28, 2007. Available at: http://www.emedicine.com/derm/topic150.htm. Accessed May 3, 2006.

33. Leyden JJ, McGinley KJ, Mills OH, et al. Propionibacterium levels in patients with and without acne vulgaris. J Invest Dermatol 1975;65:382–4.

34. Esterly NB, Furey NL, Flanagan LE. The effect of antimicrobial agents on leukocyte chemotaxis. J Invest Dermatol 1978;70:51–5.

35. Webster GF, Leyden JJ, McGinley KJ, et al. Suppression of polymorphonuclear leukocyte chemotactic factor production in Propionibacterium acnes by subminimal inhibitory concentrations of tetracycline, ampicillin, minocycline, and erythromycin. Antimicrob Agents Chemother 1982;21:770–2.

36. Jain A, Sangal L, Basal E, et al. Anti-inflammatory effects of erythromycin and tetracycline on Propionibacterium acnes induced production of chemotactic factors and reactive oxygen species by human neutrophils. Dermatol Online J 2002;8:2.

37. Webster GF, McGinley KJ, Leyden JJ. Inhibition of lipase production in Propionibacterium acnes by sub-minimal-inhibitory concentrations of tetracycline and erythromycin. Br J Dermatol 1981;104:453–7.

38. Leyden JJ. The evolving role of Propionibacterium acnes in acne. Semin Cutan Med Surg 2001;20:139–43.

39. Webster GF, Toso SM, Hegemann L. Inhibition of a model of in vitro granuloma formation by tetracyclines and ciprofloxacin. Involvement of protein kinase C. Arch Dermatol 1994;130:748–52.

40. Eady EA, Gloor M, Leyden JJ. Propionibacterium acnes resistance: a worldwide problem. Dermatology 2003;206:54–6.

41. Coates P, Vyakrnam S, Eady EA, et al. Prevalence of antibiotic-resistant propionibacteria on the skin of acne patients: 10-year surveillance data and snapshot distribution study. Br J Dermatol 2002;146:840–8.

42. Eady EA, Cove JH, Holland KT, et al. Erythromycin resistant propionibacteria in antibiotic treated acne patients: association with therapeutic failure. Br J Dermatol 1989;121:51–7.

43. Leyden JJ. Antibiotic resistant acne. Cutis 1976;17:593–606.

44. Cooper AJ. Systematic review of Propionibacterium acnes resistance to systemic antibiotics. Med J Aust 1998;169:259–61.

45. Tan HH, Goh CL, Yeo MG, et al. Antibiotic sensitivity of Propionibacterium acnes isolates from patients with acne vulgaris in a tertiary dermatological

referral centre in Singapore. Ann Acad Med Singa-pore 2001;30:22–5.

46. Dreno B, Reynaud A, Moyse D, et al. Erythromycin-resistance of cutaneous bacterial flora in acne. Eur J Dermatol 2001;11:549–53.

47. Ross JI, Snelling AM, Carnegie E, et al. Antibiotic-resistant acne: lessons from Europe. Br J Dermatol 2003;148:467–78.

48. Cunliffe WJ, Holland KT, Bojar R, et al. A randomized, double-blind comparison of a clindamycin phos-phate/benzoyl peroxide gel formulation and a match-ing clindamycin gel with respect to microbiologic activity and clinical efficacy in the topical treatment of acne vulgaris. Clin Ther 2002;24:1117–33.

49. Leyden JJ, McGinley KJ, Cavalieri S, et al. *Propioni-bacterium acnes* resistance to antibiotics in acne patients. J Am Acad Dermatol 1983;8:41–5.

50. Shalita AR, Myers JA, Krochmal L, Clindamycin Foam Study Group, et al. The safety and efficacy of clindamycin phosphate foam 1% versus clinda-mycin phosphate topical gel 1% for the treatment of acne vulgaris. J Drugs Dermatol 2005;4:48–56.

51. Thiboutot D. Acne: 1991–2001. J Am Acad Dermatol 2002;47:109–17.

52. Leyden J, Levy S. The development of antibiotic resistance in *Propionibacterium acnes*. Cutis 2001; 67(Suppl 2):21–4.

53. Ellis CN, Leyden J, Katz HI, et al. Therapeutic stud-ies with a new combination benzoyl peroxide/clinda-mycin topical gel in acne vulgaris. Cutis 2001; 67(Suppl 2):13–20.

54. Leyden JJ. Current issues in antimicrobial therapy for the treatment of acne. J Eur Acad Dermatol Venereol 2001;15(Suppl 3):51–5.

55. Shalita AR, Smith EB, Bauer E. Topical erythromycin v clindamycin therapy for acne. a multicenter, double-blind comparison. Arch Dermatol 1984;120:351–5.

56. Gollnick H, Cunliffe W, Berson D, et al. Global alliance to improve outcomes in acne. Management of acne: a report from a Global alliance to improve outcomes in acne. J Am Acad Dermatol 2003; 49(Suppl 1):S1–37.

57. Lookingbill DP, Chalker DK, Lindholm JS, et al. Treat-ment of acne with a combination clindamycin/ben-zoyl peroxide gel compared with clindamycin gel, benzoyl peroxide gel and vehicle gel: combined results of two double-blind investigations. J Am Acad Dermatol 1997;37:590–5.

58. Harkaway KS, McGinley KJ, Foglia AN, et al. Antibi-otic resistance patterns in coagulase-negative staphylococci after treatment with topical erythromy-cin, benzoyl peroxide, and combination therapy. Br J Dermatol 1992;126:586–90.

59. Thiboutot DM, Shalita AR, Yamauchi PS, et al. Adapalene gel, 0.1%, as maintenance therapy for acne vulgaris: a randomized, controlled, investiga-tor-blind follow-up of a recent combination study. Arch Dermatol 2006;142:597–602.

60. Leyden JJ, Thiboutot DM, Shalita AR, et al. Compar-ison of tazarotene and minocycline maintenance therapies in acne vulgaris. Arch Dermatol 2006; 142:605–12.

61. Leyden JJ, Kaidbey K, Gans EH. The antimicrobial effect in vivo of minocycline, doxycycline, and tetra-cycline. J Dermatolog Treat 1996;7:223–5.

62. Solodyn [package insert]. Scottsdale (AZ): Medicis Pharmaceutical Corporation; 2006.

63. Coates P, Vyakrnam S, Ravenscroft JC, et al. Efficacy of oral isotretinoin in the control of skin and nasal colonization by antibiotic-resistant propio-nibacteria in patients with acne. Br J Dermatol 2005; 153:1126–36.

64. Vowels BR, Feingold DS, Sloughfy C, et al. Effects of topical erythromycin on ecology of aerobic cutane-ous bacterial flora. Antimicrob Agents Chemother 1996;40:598–604.

65. Mills O, Thornsberry C, Cardin CW, et al. Bacterial resistance and therapeutic outcome following three months of topical acne therapy with 2% erythromy-cin gel versus its vehicle. Acta Derm Venereol 2002;82:260–5.

66. Margolis DJ, Bowe WP, Hoffstad O, et al. Antibiotic treatment of acne may be associated with upper respiratory tract infections. Arch Dermatol 2005; 141:1132–6.

67. Levy RM, Huang EY, Roling D, et al. Effect of antibi-otics on the oropharyngeal flora in patients with acne. Arch Dermatol 2003;139:467–71.

68. Adams SJ, Cunliffe WJ, Cooke EM. Long-term anti-biotic therapy for acne vulgaris: effects on the bowel flora of patients and their relatives. J Invest Dermatol 1985;85:35–7.

69. Miller YW, Eady EA, Lacey RW, et al. Sequential antibiotic therapy for acne promotes the carriage of resistant staphylococci on the skin of contacts. J Antimicrob Chemother 1996;38:829–37.

A Current Review of Topical Benzoyl Peroxide: New Perspectives on Formulation and Utilization

Emil A. Tanghetti, MD[a,b,*], Karl F. Popp, RPh[c]

KEYWORDS

- Benzoyl peroxide • Topical use • Acne
- Combination therapy • Antibacterial resistance

Sales of over-the-counter benzoyl peroxide (BPO) are currently approaching $1 billion annually, effectively securing its position as the most widely used topical acne medication in dermatology. Its safety and efficacy are unquestionable. Because it has been many years since this product was thoroughly reviewed in the literature, this article provides the most recent perspectives regarding the topical use of BPO in dermatology.

BPO is an organic peroxide consisting of white crystal agglomerates that are soluble in chloroform and other organic solvents but insoluble in water.[1] Although stable at room temperature, it is flammable[2] and is explosive when heated to temperatures of greater than 100°C.[3]

Although a powerful oxidizing agent, it is nontoxic to humans and is used in food processing to bleach flour and oils and in various industrial applications.[1] BPO, derived from a byproduct of coal tar, was used as early as 1905 as a nonirritating oxidizing antiseptic. Although BPO was mainly used as a bleach for flour in the first part of the 20th century, dermatologists also prescribed it for wound healing and treating burns and chronic skin ulcers.[4]

PHARMACOKINETIC AND SAFETY PROFILE

A study by Nacht and colleagues[5] examined BPO penetration through normal skin and its systemic disposition. A study of radiolabelled BPO penetration through excised human skin found that under maximal steady state conditions, 4.5% of the applied dose was delivered to the skin in an 8-hour period. Of the total amount of BPO applied topically, 95.5% was recovered unchanged from the skin at 8 hours. Topically applied BPO was found to penetrate unchanged through the stratum corneum or into the follicles. It then diffused into the epidermis and dermis, where it is converted to benzoic acid, possibly with the aid of follicular bacteria. Systemically, studies in primates showed that benzoic acid is absorbed as benzoate and excreted unchanged in the urine. BPO seems to avoid degradation by the liver.[5]

Haustein[6] studied 100 patients aged 12–28 years who had acne treated with 10% BPO gel twice daily for 8 weeks. Before treatment, they were tested with BPO 5%, 1%, and 0.1% embedded in paraffin for 24 hours, and results were read at 24, 48, and 72 hours. Of the 100 patients, only

a Department of Dermatology, University of California at Davis, Davis, CA, USA
b Center for Dermatology and Laser Surgery, Sacramento, CA, USA
c 1775 Duck Pond Road, Schodack Landing, NY 12156, USA
* Corresponding author.
E-mail address: smoore@physicianresources.org (E.A. Tanghetti).

Dermatol Clin 27 (2009) 17–24
doi:10.1016/j.det.2008.07.001

2 reacted to the BPO 1%, whereas the 0.1% test concentration gave only a questionable reaction. These results suggest that BPO is a weak allergen and is more likely to give an irritant reaction, especially at higher concentrations.

Six patients (6%) complained of stinging, itching, burning and erythema, edema, dryness, and desquamation at treatment initiation. These symptoms disappeared in 5 patients with continued use, including after a short break. In addition to these study findings, clinical experience suggests that BPO, at the concentrations usually used in practice, is most often associated with irritant reactions that often resolve with a drug holiday. True contact dermatitis can occur but is relatively uncommon. These studies highlight the importance of the delivery systems and vehicles used in clinical practice.

ANTIBACTERIAL AND ANTI-INFLAMMATORY PROPERTIES OF BENZOYL PEROXIDE IN ACNE

BPO has been shown to have numerous modes of activity. This remarkable drug has been shown to possess antimicrobial and anti-inflammatory,[7] keratolytic,[8] and wound-healing activity.[9,10] How BPO affects sebum secretion rate remains controversial.[11–14] However, current thinking maintains that no topical agents are sebostatic.[15,16]

Antimicrobial Activity

Over the years BPO activity in acne has been shown to be caused by antimicrobial activity that is rapid and bacteriostatic and possibly bactericidal.[15] In 1974, Fulton and colleagues[17] compared the antibacterial activity of BPO and vitamin A acid. They noted that BPO "is more than just another epidermal irritant; it is also a potent bacteriostat."[17] They also noted that the vehicle is critical. In the alcohol gels studied, residual deposition of BPO on the skin after the alcohol vehicle evaporated allowed continued contact.

In vivo studies comparing *Corynebacterium acnes* recovery from sebum in 10 subjects applying BPO 10% in alcohol gel vehicle twice daily and vehicle twice daily found a marked reduction in bacteria in the sebum of those using active treatment (Bollinger JN, Rowlands JR, Gause EM, personal communication). This group found that BPO also decreased the ratio of free fatty acids to free esters in sebum. Currently, the role of free fatty acids in acne pathogenesis is no longer considered important.[1]

A study by Cove and Holland[18] in 1981, examined survival curves of 8 different microorganisms known to colonize skin in the presence of BPO. The microorganisms varied in increasing sensitivity to BPO as follows: *Propionibacterium acnes, Staphylococcus capitis, S epidermis, S hominis, P avidum, P granulosum,* and the yeast *Pityrosporum ovale.* BPO had a homogenous bactericidal effect, suggesting that no resistant subpopulations were present. The authors point out that BPO exerts its bactericidal activity through oxidation, leading to the release of highly reactive oxygen intermediates that oxidize proteins in bacterial cell membranes.[18]

A study using high-pressure liquid chromatography 1 to 2 minutes after application of BPO emulsion to the skin found that BPO rapidly penetrates the stratum corneum. Additionally, BPO is degraded to benzoic acid, leaving no detectable BPO depot in the stratum corneum.[19]

Burkhart and Burkhart[20] showed that *P acnes* are capable of secreting protective biofilm polysaccharides, which may explain some of the difficulty of delivering effective levels of antimicrobials within the skin. BPO, with its oxidative properties, appears to have a role in destroying this biofilm. This biofilm model helps to illustrate the use of BPO in facilitating the delivery of topical antibiotics and other agents to the targeted bacteria.[20,21]

Although this biofilm model is intriguing, the clusters of *P acne* and other bacteria are encased in a matrix of sebum and keratin, which acts as a barrier to the delivery of therapeutic products as well as provides for an anaerobic environment. Here again, the oxidative and keratalytic properties of BPO provide utility in weakening this protective barrier. Perhaps the final word and summary of the current data on the antibacterial efficacy of BPO in acne should go to Kligman,[22] who declared in 1995 that "No prescription antibiotic can begin to match the antibacterial efficacy of benzoyl peroxide. Twice-daily applications for five days will reduce the *P acnes* population by more than 95%! Moreover, unlike the case with topical antibiotics, *P acnes* has not been smart enough to evolve resistance to benzoyl peroxide."

Keratolytic Activity

An important and often overlooked property of BPO is its effect on comedonal acne. A study by Waller and colleagues[8] compared the keratolytic efficacy and cutaneous barrier disruption of BPO 2%, retinoic acid 0.05%, and salicylic acid 2%, a well-established keratolytic. Sites on untreated volar forearms of volunteers were treated under occlusion and unoccluded and examined at 3 and 6 hours. At 3 hours, BPO was significantly more keratolytic, as shown by the amount of stratum corneum removed with tape stripping.

Transepidermal water loss (TEWL) was used to study barrier disruption, which was found to correlate with the depth of stratum corneum removal. Salicylic acid had the greatest keratolytic activity at more superficial depths.

Perhaps because of the vehicle used in this study, BPO was more effective and created a higher TEWL effect at deeper layers. This effect was seen as a complement to its known antibacterial efficacy. The authors also note that the ability of BPO to disrupt the stratum corneum barrier may improve penetration of drugs that are coadministered.[8]

CLINICAL STUDY REVIEW
Benzoyl Peroxide Monotherapy

The first use of BPO in the management of acne was reported by Canadian dermatologist William Pace,[23] who identified it as the active ingredient in a chlorhydroxyquinolin ointment in a petrolatum base (Quinolor Compound Ointment, ER Squibb and Sons). After discussing BPO solubility issues with John King, Pace then consulted a London, Ontario pharmacist, Clare Munro, and incorporated the solution of BPO to a commercial cream base (Dermabase, Borden, Ltd., Don Mills, Ontario, Canada). This pharmacy-compounded product was reported by Pace to be as effective as the original but much less irritating, and formulated into an aesthetically acceptable, clinically efficacious acne treatment.

The effectiveness of Pace's cream came to the attention of Werner Stiefel who commercialized BPO for the treatment of acne. Stiefel, who was educated as a chemical engineer, engaged the team of Cox and Ciufo,[24] who created and patented a stable composition of BPO for the treatment of acne.

Since then, many BPO antiacne products have been marketed. Dosage forms include gels, cream, lotions, aerosols, foams, wipes, pads, masks, and solutions. Concentrations have varied from around 1% to as high as 20%. Various drug delivery systems have also been used with BPO, including micronization, polymeric drug release, encapsulation, entrapment, particle coating, cosolvent systems, combinations with other actives, combinations of actives to address different therapeutic needs, and copackaging with companion products.

From the regimen of sulfur with BPO and then onto combinations with salicylic acid, sunscreens, antibiotics, and barrier repair agents, dermatologists have recognized that treatment of skin conditions often requires combination therapy to address the multifaceted causes seen in skin disease. Inventors and companies have been searching for the utopian treatment for acne, but to no avail. Efforts have been directed toward addressing the technical deficiencies that are common with BPO products.

Skin irritation is the main issue observed by patients and physicians when BPO is used to treat acne. Irritation potential may be reduced through micronizing the BPO particle or making it softer and less abrasive. Other additives, such as emollients, polymers, and anti-irritants, may be included in the compositions to improve the product's aesthetics. Furthermore, the rate of release of the drug and physical availability of the active may also be modified through drug delivery approaches, such as encapsulation, coating technologies, and entrapment.

Although early BPO products such as BenzaGel, Panoxyl, Desquam, and Persagel served dermatology well, they were essentially replaced with newer delivery systems. A product based on dimethyl isosorbide as a solvent for BPO was developed by dermatologist Richard DeVillez.[25] Seeing the need for the active to penetrate better, DeVillez found that BPO dissolved in dimethyl isosorbide and that stability could be maintained in these compositions. Won and colleagues[26] found that BPO could be entrapped in a porous styrene–divinylbenzene polymer structure, which is now known as microsponge technology. Both delivery systems reduced irritation.

Flynn[27] recognized the need to remove excess skin oils found around acne lesions and found fumed silica served this purpose. This concept became a major part of the Oxy acne franchise.

Cox and Ciufo, Young, Fulton, and Klein and Fox each contributed to the knowledge used to produce stable BPO compositions today.[24,28–30] Cox[24] recognized that having BPO at least partially suspended improved stability. He coupled this with the inclusion of an organic emollient and the reduction of the particle size of the drug crystal. Young[28] pioneered a hydroalcoholic gel that used polyoxyethylene-based surfactants to reduce product drag during application. Fulton[29] showed that using a high concentration of a polar emollient, glycerin, also resulted in not only a stable composition but also one perceived to be nonirritating. Klein and Fox[30] further found that stability improved if a small amount of dioctyl sodium sulfosuccinate was added to the formulation.

A new BPO product in a novel solvent-based system has been formulated that apparently, similar to those containing dimethyl isosorbide, has the ability to solubilize BPO and facilitate a rapid and more complete absorption of the BPO. Results of two recent trials suggest a more rapid response in treating comedones with similar efficacy in treating inflammatory lesions to a 5 percent water-based benzyl peroxide/clindamycin combination. This new solvent system did show a significant increase in stinging, burning, erythema, and dryness during the first two weeks. It is possible that the volatile agents in this product are also solubilizing the lipids in the comedones, resulting in an unusually rapid response for comedonal acne.

There are an incredible number of new and old benzyl peroxide products available today. There are many differences in these formulations, which could have a significant effect on delivery tolerability and efficacy. Well-designed head-to-head studies that evaluate these products in a prospective manner are lacking. Therefore, it is difficult for comparative assessments on safety or efficacy across these different formulations to be made.

A single-blind comparison of the safety and efficacy of twice-daily BPO 4% gel and once-daily adapalene 0.1% gel showed that both treatments were similarly effective in treating comedonal and inflammatory lesions after 11 weeks. However, BPO 4% was statistically superior to adapalene 0.1% in the percentage reduction of all lesions at weeks two and five ($P = .0007$ and $P = .0944$, respectively). This difference is important because patients who have acne typically comply better with therapy if they see a rapid response. The similar effects of both BPO and adapalene on comedones in this study highlights the importance of BPOs in the treatment of this form of acne. In fact, the consensus groups' opinion does not even mention this class of products in the initial treatment of comedonal acne. Hopefully, renewed attention on this subject will permit a better appreciation of this point. Experts suggested that in BPO–retinoid combination therapy, the rapid upfront response to BPO compensated for the retinoid's later onset of action both for inflammatory and comedonal acne.[31]

In a comparison of 6% BPO gel and 1% clindamycin phosphate lotion, the BPO gel produced more rapid and significantly greater reductions in *P acnes* counts ($P < .01$) and fluorescence.[32]

The current trend in the management of acne is to combine BPO with other medications that have a different mode of action.[15] However, BPO monotherapy is still used particularly in the form of washes designed to be rinsed off rather than remain on the skin where they may be irritating. These washes are increasingly available in different strengths and various cleansing bases for patients with sensitive or irritation-prone skin. Experts have suggested that exposing the skin to an acne treatment is more important than the duration of exposure or the medication

concentration. However, data supporting this in large controlled clinical trials are lacking. The authors' believe that leave-on products with slow-release BPO designed for longer skin contact are potentially more effective in affecting a positive clinical outcome.

Burkhart[33] suggested that the rapid effect of BPO washes may be from the ability of the BPO radicals to react with bacterial membranes and intracellular organelles within milliseconds of application. This approach may be especially effective, because overzealous washing and scrubbing of acne lesions may actually worsen the disease and increase irritation.[33,34]

Occlusive moisturizers act as an emollient to provide rapid repair of the skin barrier.[35] Occlusives alone are effective, but inefficient and not cosmetically acceptable. A humectant alone may exacerbate transepidermal water loss.[35] Occlusive agents, such as dimethicone, are designed to help prevent water evaporation, and glycerin, which is a humectant, attracts water from the dermis to the epidermis. These formulations combining a humectant with an emollient assist with rehydration and restoration of the epidermal defensive. Another strategy for improving the tolerability of BPO is to formulate it in a 10% urea base, which might moisturize the skin because of its humectant property[36] and add to its antiacne efficacy because of its keratolytic activity.[37]

Combination Therapy

Benzoyl peroxide and topical antibiotics

The success of both BPO and topical antibiotics in acne treatment prompted many studies of their combination to increase efficacy through combining drugs with differing but complementary modes of activity. Moreover, well-designed combination therapy may take advantage of the possible synergy between the effects of the agents chosen.[38] However, as *P acnes* resistance to topical and oral antibiotics began to increase worldwide, strategies were sought to minimize this threat. Topical combination therapy is prescribed using separate products, with many combinations, such as BPO with clindamycin or erythromycin, used to increase efficacy and decrease risk for resistance.[39,40]

In 1985, Klein's patent for the first combination of BPO with an antibiotic, erythromycin, was issued and with it came the birth of a product compounded by the pharmacist and dispensed to the patient (Benzamycin Topical Gel, Dermik). This product was to be refrigerated by the patient and discarded after 90 days. The next-generation product (BenzaClin Topical Gel, Dermik) is a mixture of

BPO 5% with clindamycin phosphate 1% that is similarly compounded by the pharmacist and can remain at room temperature for 90 days, after which it should be discarded by the patient. Another factory-blended BPO 5%/clindamycin phosphate 1% gel (Duac Topical Gel, Stiefel Laboratories) is available in a composition that is refrigerated by the distribution channel and then kept at room temperature by the patient for 60 days, after which it should be discarded. All of these products have been shown to be widely accepted by physicians and patients.

The 2003 acne treatment consensus guidelines state that oral and topical antibiotics should not be used as monotherapy in acne because chronic use is associated with the emergence of resistant bacterial variants.[15] In a study by Cunliffe and coworkers,[41] resistant P acnes appeared as early as 8 weeks after initiation of therapy with topical clindamycin monotherapy and increased over the 16 weeks of the study. The recent Scientific Panel on Antibiotic Use in Dermatology convened to evaluate the use of antibiotics in dermatology.[42]

Prolonged topical or oral antibiotic therapy for acne vulgaris is best accompanied by the use of BPO to optimize efficacy and mitigate the emergence of less-sensitive P acnes strains. The presence of less-sensitive P acnes organisms may contribute to decreased efficacy of antibiotic treatment in some patients, especially if a high density of these strains is present. However, oral antibiotics, such as doxycycline, minocycline, and topical clindamycin, have continued to maintain efficacy in many patients, specifically when used in appropriate combination with other agents, such as BPO and topical retinoids.

The use of combination therapy with BPO to help minimize the development of resistance is important to note in clinical practice. In more than 35 years of use in acne management, bacterial resistance to BPO has not developed.[15]

Several studies have shown the combination of BPO and a topical antibiotic was more effective and better tolerated than monotherapy with either agent.[41,43–46] A BPO 5%/clindamycin 1% pharmacy-compounded water-based gel is available, as is a premixed BPO 5%/clindamycin 1% in a dimethicone- and glycerin-containing gel. These gels were proven to be safe and effective in the treatment of acne. On evaluation of the reduction of inflammatory lesions at 11 weeks, the dimethicone- and glycerin-containing BPO/clindamycin gel used once daily and the BPO/clindamycin water-based gel used twice daily yielded similar results.

Cunliffe and coworkers[41] compared clindamycin 1%/BPO 5% gel with clindamycin 1% gel monotherapy. Again, combination clindamycin/

BPO therapy produced significantly greater reductions from baseline in inflammatory lesion, total lesion, and comedone counts compared with clindamycin monotherapy ($P \leq .046$), and greater improvements in patients' and physicians' clinical global improvement scores. This study was particularly notable in showing a greater than 1600% increase in P acnes counts from baseline to week 16 in the group undergoing clindamycin monotherapy. In contrast, the group undergoing combination therapy showed decreases in resistant bacteria, which correlated with reductions in inflammatory and total lesions ($r^2 = 0.31$ and 0.28; $P = .016$ and 0.027, respectively). Both the total P acnes count and the clindamycin-resistant P acnes counts were decreased with combination therapy but not with clindamycin monotherapy.

A 2007 randomized, assessor-blind study compared the safety and efficacy of once-daily applications of topical clindamycin 1%/BPO 5% and twice-daily applications of erythromycin + zinc acetate administered for 12 weeks in 148 patients with mild to moderate acne.[47] The BPO/clindamycin combination showed an earlier onset of action; at week 1, the proportion of patients with at least a 30% reduction in non-inflammatory lesions was 31.5% for the BPO/clindamycin group and 17.3% for erythromycin/zinc. This trend continued until study end, although reductions in total lesion count were similar at termination (69.8% and 64.5%, respectively). Both treatments were well tolerated.

BENZOYL PEROXIDE AND RETINOIDS

Combination therapy with BPO and antibacterials is effective in reducing bacterial proliferation and countering inflammation. Because effects in comedonal acne have not been well described or characterized in clinical trials, it is prudent to combine BPO with topical retinoids, an already important mainstay in acne treatment with strong anticomedogenic and comedolytic activity.[7,15]

Retinoids normalize the desquamation of the follicular epithelium and prevent the formation of new comedones, the precursor to all acne lesions.[7,48] Retinoids also enhance the penetration of other topical drugs into the follicle.[8] The introduction of less-irritating retinoids and more-emollient vehicles has made this therapy extremely tolerable. For example, in a study by Shalita and colleagues,[49] a 6% BPO wash used in combination with 0.1% tretinoin microsphere reduced skin tightness compared with tretinoin monotherapy.

In another study, patients with moderate to severe acne using tazarotene 0.1% cream each evening and were randomized to morning applications of either vehicle gel or a clindamycin 1%/BPO 5% gel containing the emollient dimethicone and the humectant glycerin.[50] The retinoid plus clindamycin/BPO regimen showed a significantly greater reduction in comedonal lesions than tazarotene monotherapy beginning at week 4, and continued to be statistically significant throughout the 12-week study. Again this finding highlights the importance of benzyl peroxide in the treatment of comedonal acne. Surprisingly, clinical significance in inflammatory lesions was only seen in patients who had more than 25 lesions. The clindamycin 1%/BPO 5% gel was better tolerated and patients experienced a lower incidence of peeling and drying compared with those treated with tazarotene cream monotherapy. This finding was particularly noticeable and statistically significant at week 4 during retinization. Similar findings were also noted in a study using the same humectants- and emollient-containing BPO/clindamycin gel in combination with the retinoid adapalene.[51]

A fixed-dose, once-daily combination gel with adapalene 0.1% and BPO 2.5% was recently developed (EpiDuo, Galderma Laboratories).[52] A 12-month study enrolled 452 subjects to assess the efficacy and safety of the combination. Reductions in total, inflammatory, and comedonal lesions began as early as week one. At 12 months, when data from the last observation carried forward were examined, the median percent reductions from baseline were 65%, 70%, and 66% in total, inflammatory, and comedonal lesion counts, respectively. Treatment was well tolerated overall, with only a 2.0% dropout rate from adverse events. Studies have not compared the efficacy or tolerance of this product compared with currently used regimens of a BPO and clindamycin/retinoid combination.

SUMMARY

BPO is arguably the most widely used topical treatment for acne, with more than 35 years of safe and effective use. A resurgence in the use of this agent has recently occurred, despite the development of effective antibiotic and retinoid regimens. This resurgence seems to from the increasing appreciation of the bactericidal and anti-inflammatory capabilities and anticomedolitic properties of BPO. Most importantly, however, unlike other antibacterial products, bacterial resistance to BPO has not yet been observed and is unlikely to happen. It is generally agreed that adding BPO is a sine qua non of antibiotic treatment of acne because of its ability to reduce the risk for

resistance and its activity against both sensitive and resistant strains of *P acnes*.

Although earlier formulations of BPO were somewhat limited by irritation, new vehicles have greatly improved the tolerability of BPO monotherapy and combinations. Adding excipients such as urea and glycerin, and the emollient dimethicone to the base also improve tolerability. Intriguing new research suggests that combining BPO and antibiotics or other drugs containing tertiary amines may enhance the free radical formation believed to be the basis of BPO's bactericidal activity. Strategies such as this to boost the activity of BPO may eventually result in greatly reduced antibiotic use in managing acne.

ACKNOWLEDGEMENTS

The authors would like to acknowledge the editorial assistance of Stacey Moore at Physician Resources, LLC.

REFERENCES

1. Cotterill JA. Benzoyl peroxide. Acta Dermatovener (Stockholm) 1980;(Suppl 89):57–63.
2. Prat J. Mem, Serv Etat (Paris) 1948;34:335.
3. Dickey FH, et al. Ind and Eng Chem 1948;26:4518.
4. Merker PC. Benzoyl peroxide: a history of early research and researchers. Int J Dermatol 2002;41:185–8.
5. Nacht S, Yeung D, Beasley JN, et al. Benzoyl peroxide: percutaneous penetration and metabolic disposition. J Am Acad Dermatol 1981;4:31–7.
6. Haustein U-F, Tegetmeyer L, Ziegler V. Allergic and irritant potential of benzoyl peroxide. Contact Dermatitis 1985;13:252–7.
7. Gollnick GH, Schramm M. Topical drug treatment in acne. Dermatology 1998;196:119–25.
8. Waller JM, Dreher F, Behnam S, et al. 'Keratolytic' properties of benzoyl peroxide and retinoic acid resemble salicylic acid in man. Skin Pharmacol Physiol 2006;19:283–9.
9. Fanta D, Bardach H, Poitscheck C. Investigations of the bacteriostatic effect of benzoyl peroxide. Arch Dermatol Res 1979;264:369–71.
10. Alvarez OM, Mertz PM, Eaglstein WH. Benzoyl peroxide and epidermal wound healing. Arch Dermatol 1983;119:222–5.
11. Cunliffe WJ, Stainton C, Forster RA. Topical benzoyl peroxide increases the sebum excretion rate in patients with acne. Br J Dermatol 1983;109:577–9.
12. Schmidt JB, Neumann R, Knobler R, et al. Sebum suppression by benzoylperoxide. Dermatologica 1985;170:165–9.
13. Gloor M, Klump H, Wirth H. Cytokinetic studies on the sebo-suppressive effect of drugs using the

example of benzoyl peroxide. Arch Dermatol Res 1980;267:97–9.

14. Burkhart CG, Butcher C, Burkhart CN, et al. Effects of benzoyl peroxide on lipogenesis in sebaceous glands using an animal model. J Cutan Med Surg 2000;4:138–41.

15. Gollnick H, Cunliffe W, Berson D, et al. Management of acne. A report from a global alliance to improve outcomes in acne. J Am Acad Dermatol 2003;49:S1–38.

16. Stinco G, Bragadin G, Trotter D, et al. Relationship between sebostatic activity, tolerability and efficacy of three topical drugs to treat mild to moderate acne. J Eur Acad Dermatol Venereol. 2007;21:320–5.

17. Fulton JK, Farzad-Bakshandeh A, Bradley S. Studies on the mechanism of action of topical benzoyl peroxide and vitamin A acid in acne vulgaris. J Cutan Pathol. 1974;1:191–200.

18. Cove H, Holland KT. The effect of benzoyl peroxide on cutaneous micro-organisms in vitro. J Appl Bacteriol 1983;54:379–82.

19. Seubert S, Seubert A, Ippen H. Penetration of benzoyl peroxide in the skin [in German]. Hautarzt 1984;35:455–8.

20. Burkhart CN, Burkhart CG. Genome sequence of Propionibacterium acnes reveals immunogenic and surface-associated genes confirming existence of the acne biofilm. Int J Dermatol. 2006;45:872.

21. Burkhart CN, Burkhart CG. Microbiology's principle of biofilms as a major factor in the pathogenesis of acne vulgaris. Int J Dermatol 2003;42:925–7.

22. Kligman AM. Acne vulgaris: tricks and treatments. Part II: The benzoyl peroxide saga. Cutis 1995;56:260–1.

23. Pace WE. A benzoyl peroxide-sulfur cream for acne vulgaris. Can Med Assoc J 1965;93:252–4.

24. Cox RM, Ciufo LR, inventors; Stiefel Laboratories, Inc, assignee. Stable benzoyl peroxide composition. US patent 3 535 422. October 20, 1970.

25. DeVillez RL, inventor; Board of Regents, The University of Texas System, assignee. Therapeutic compositions containing benzoyl peroxide. US patent 4 923 900. May 8, 1990.

26. Won R, inventor; Advanced Polymer Systems, Inc, assignee. Method for delivery an active ingredient by controlled release utilizing a novel delivery vehicle which can be prepared by a process utilizing the active ingredient as a porogen. US patent 4 690 825. September 1, 1985.

27. Flynn RG, Pitkin CG, Hileman GA, inventors; Norcliff Thayer, Inc, assignee. Use of fumed silica for treating oily skin and acne. US patent 4 536 399. August 20, 1985.

28. Young HY, inventor; Stiefel Laboratories, Inc, assignee. Therapeutic composition. US patent 4 056 611. November 1, 1977.

29. Fulton JE Jr, inventor; AHC Pharmacal, Inc, assignee. Composition and method for the treatment of acne. US patent 4 189 501. February 19, 1980.

30. Klein RW, Foxx ME, inventors; Dermik Laboratories, Inc, assignee. Stable benzoyl peroxide composition. US patent 4 387 107. June 7, 1983.

31. do Nascimento LV, Guedes ACM, Magalhaes GM, et al. Single-blind and comparative clinical study of the efficacy and safety of benzoyl peroxide 4% gel (BID) and adapalene 0.1% gel (QD) in the treatment of acne vulgaris. J Dermatolog Treat 2003;14:166–71.

32. Gans EH, Kligman AM. Comparative efficacy of clindamycin and benzoyl peroxide for in vivo suppression of Propionibacterium acnes. J Dermatolog Treat 2002;13:101–10.

33. Burkhart CG, Scheinfeld NS. Benzoyl peroxide skin washes: basis, logic, effectiveness and tolerance. Skinmed November-December, 2005, 370.

34. Mills OH Jr, Kligman AM. Acne detergicans. Arch Dermatol 1975;111:65–8.

35. Draelos ZD. Concepts in skin care maintenance. Cutis 2005;76:S19–25.

36. Grace K, Sattar H, Baker H. Urea and retinoic acid in ichthyosis and their effect on transepidermal water loss and water holding capacity of stratum corneum. Acta Dermatovenereol (Stockholm) 1973;53:114–8.

37. Swanbeck G. A new treatment for ichthyosis and other hyperkeratotic conditions. Acta Dermatovenereol (Stockholm) 1968;48:123–7.

38. Leyden J. Introduction to: are 2 combined antimicrobial mechanisms better than 1 for the treatment of acne vulgaris? Cutis 2001;67:5–7.

39. Eady EA, Farmery MR, Ross JI, et al. Effects of benzoyl peroxide and erythromycin alone and in combination against antibiotic-sensitive and -resistant skin bacteria from acne patients. Br J Dermatol 1994;131:331–6.

40. Eady EA, Bojar RA, Jones CE, et al. The effects of acne treatment with a combination of benzoyl peroxide and erythromycin on skin carriage of erythromycin-resistant propionibacteria. Br J Dermatol 1996;134:107–13.

41. Cunliffe WJ, Holland KT, Bojar R, et al. A randomized, double-blind comparison of a clindamycin phosphate/benzoyl peroxide gel formulation and a matching clindamycin gel with respect to microbiologic activity and clinical efficacy in the topical treatment of acne vulgaris. Clin Ther 2002;24:1117–33.

42. Leyden JJ, Del Rosso JQ, Webster GF. Clinical considerations in the treatment of acne vulgaris and other inflammatory skin disorders: focus on antibiotic resistance. Cutis. 2007;79(Suppl 6):9–25.

43. Lookingbill DP, Chalker DK, Lindholm JS, et al. Treatment of acne with a combination clindamycin/benzoyl peroxide gel compared with clindamycin gel, benzoyl peroxide gel, and vehicle gel: combined results of two double-blind investigations. J Am Acad Dermatol 1997;37:590–5.

44. Leyden JJ, Hickman JG, Jarratt MT, et al. The efficacy and safety of a combination benzoyl peroxide/clindamycin topical gel compared with benzoyl peroxide alone and a benzoyl erythromycin combination product. J Cutan Med Surg 2001;5:37–42.

45. Tschen E, Jones T. A new treatment for acne vulgaris combining benzoyl peroxide with clindamycin. J Drugs Dermatol 2002;2:153–7.

46. Jansen T, Korber A, Folkmann A, et al. Topical acne therapy with a combination of clindamycin 1% and benzoyl peroxide 5%. Akt Dermatol 2005;31:566–71.

47. Langner A, Sheehan-Dare R, Layton A. A randomized, single-blind comparison of topical clindamycin + benzoyl peroxide (Duac®) and erythromycin + zinc acetate (Zineryt®) in the treatment of mild to moderate facial acne vulgaris. J Eur Acad Dermatol Venereol 2007;21:311–9.

48. Leyden JJ. A review of the use of combination therapies for the treatment of acne vulgaris. J Am Acad Dermatol 2003;49:S200–10.

49. Shalita AR, Rafal ES, Anderson DN, et al. Compared efficacy and safety of tretinoin 0.1% microsphere gel alone and in combination with benzoyl peroxide 6% cleanser for the treatment of acne vulgaris. Cutis 2003;72:167–72.

50. Tanghetti E, Abramovits W, Solomon B, et al. Tazarotene versus tazarotene plus clindamycin/benzoyl peroxide in the treatment of acne vulgaris: a multicenter, double blind, randomized parallel group trial. J Drugs Dermatol 2006;5:256–61.

51. Del Rosso JQ. Study results of benzoyl peroxide 5%/clindamycin 1% topical gel, adapalene 0.1% gel, and use in combination for acne vulgaris. J Drugs Dermatol 2007;6:616–22.

52. Pariser DM, Westmoreland P, Morris A, et al. Long-term safety and efficacy of a unique fixed-dose combination of gel of adapalene 0.01% and benzoyl peroxide 2.5% for the treatment of acne vulgaris. J Drugs Dermatol 2007;6:899–905.

Topical Antibiotics in Dermatology: Emerging Patterns of Resistance

Dirk M. Elston, MD

KEYWORDS

• Bacterial • Resistance • Skin • Acne • Infection

Topical agents are widely used to treat skin conditions. The skin is readily accessible and topical agents can be applied at high concentration, achieving effective levels locally with little systemic toxicity. The high local levels of antibiotic that can be achieved with topical formulations can help kill bacteria in bacterial biofilms.[1] Resistance to topical antibiotics is of growing concern to dermatologists. The armamentarium of topical agents is limited, and those that are available cannot afford to be lost. Responsible use of topical antibiotics will preserve their efficacy. This article focuses on evidence of emerging resistance, the implications to clinical practice, and strategies to minimize occurrence.

TOPICAL ANTIBIOTICS TO ELIMINATE COLONIZATION

Responsible use of antibiotics will preserve their efficacy as therapeutic agents. Oral and topical antibiotics have been used to reduce postoperative infections, but evidence suggests that only a brief course of preoperative antibiotic is needed and that adding a topical agent provides little benefit. Although a single dose of preoperative antibiotic can reduce postoperative infections, prophylactic regimens exceeding 48 hours provide no added benefit.[2] Adding antibiotic to the local anesthetic is an effective alternative, with less potential to alter resident flora or induce resistance.

White petrolatum is suitable for postoperative wound care. A randomized, double-blind, prospective trial comparing white petrolatum with bacitracin ointment in postprocedure care of 1249 wounds showed a slightly higher rate of infection in the petrolatum group (nine in the white petrolatum group versus four in the bacitracin group). The difference was not statistically significant. All but one of the infections in the white petrolatum group were caused by *Staphylococcus aureus*, whereas those in the bacitracin group were more likely to be gram-negative and require more expensive therapy ($P = .004$). Four patients developed allergic contact dermatitis from bacitracin.[3] Together these data question the value of topical antibiotics for routine postoperative wound care and suggest that white petrolatum may be preferable.

Colonization with methicillin-resistant *Staphylococcus aureus* (MRSA) is appropriate to address in some situations. Because oral and intravenous antibiotics used for MRSA infections achieve poor levels on the skin surface, topical agents such as chlorhexidine, triclosan, or Dakin's solution (dilute bleach) have been used to address surface colonization. Commonly used oral antibiotics, such as sulfa drugs and doxycycline, also achieve poor levels in the nares. Clindamycin achieves good levels in the nares but resistance is increasing. Because oral therapy is problematic in nasal carriage, topical agents are often used. Sites of colonization should be addressed globally, because addressing nasal carriage alone has little effect.[4] Whole-body washing with chlorhexidine reduces skin colonization but is most effective as part of a global approach addressing the gastrointestinal tract, wounds, and nares.[5]

Perioperative prophylaxis with nasal mupirocin and topical triclosan for 5 days has been shown

The author has no relevant conflict of interest, but has been a consultant for Abbott, Medicis, and Collagenix.
Department of Dermatology, Geisinger Medical Center, 100 North Academy Avenue, Danville, PA 17821, USA
E-mail address: dmelston@geisinger.edu

Dermatol Clin 27 (2009) 25–31
doi:10.1016/j.det.2008.07.004

to reduce the incidence of MRSA infection after orthopaedic and vascular surgery. Although mupirocin resistance is increasing, it remained effective in one study spanning 4 years.[6] Screening for MRSA and decolonization with topical antiseptics on admission to an intensive care unit (ICU) has been shown to reduce rates of MRSA infection when combined with effective barrier precautions. In one study, topical agents were used in the nose along with daily bed baths with 4% chlorhexidine. These interventions resulted in a threefold reduction in the proportion of patients who had MRSA ($P = .005$) and a decrease in mean length of stay ($P < .001$).[7]

In a randomized controlled trial, 74% of patients treated with a chlorhexidine gluconate wash plus intranasal mupirocin, rifampin, and doxycycline showed sustained clearing (≥ 3 months) compared with 32% of those who underwent no treatment ($P = .0001$). At 8 months, 54% of the treated patients still had negative cultures and the difference remained statistically significant ($P < .0001$). Mupirocin-resistant strains were associated with treatment failure ($P = .0003$), but most resistant strains were already present at baseline. During therapy, mupirocin resistance emerged in only 5% of isolates.[8]

Failure may represent recolonization rather than a failure to clear the initial colonization. In a study of 87 MRSA-positive health care workers, topical antibiotics and antiseptics resulted in clearing of 7 individuals (84%). MRSA was detected only in later nasopharyngeal swabs in 11 of 14 individuals who remained colonized, suggesting recolonization. Further screening identified nasal colonization of household contacts in 8 of the 11 patients.[9]

Chlorhexidine has good activity against staphylococcal isolates, including those resistant to iodophor.[10,11] Chlorhexidine is less active against MRSA compared with methicillin-sensitive staphylococci (MSSA) ($P = . 017$), but its activity can be improved when it is delivered in an alcoholic vehicle.[12] The ethanol alone has significant antibacterial activity.[13] Povidone iodine seems to be equally active against MRSA and MSSA strains, including those with decreased sensitivity to chlorhexidine.[14] MRSA isolates have emerged that show resistance to both chlorhexidine and quaternary ammonium compounds (including benzalkonium chloride).[15] Triclosan resistance is emerging in both MSSA and MRSA strains.[16,17] Over-the-counter availability and widespread use contributes to the spread of resistance, and increasing resistance to common biocides has been documented over time.[18] Some resistance is plasmid-mediated and may spread among isolates.[19,20]

Silver sulfadiazine 1%, mupirocin 2%, and fusidic acid 2% all show antistaphylococcal activity and are similarly effective in reducing local burn wound bacterial count and preventing systemic infection in an animal model of MRSA infection.[21] Fusidic acid–resistance is spreading and has become a significant problem in some countries.[22]

MUPIROCIN RESISTANCE

Mupirocin resistance is emerging as a significant problem and has been reported in as many as 50% of isolates.[23] Fortunately, the rates are generally much lower, but continued surveillance is essential. A Canadian study of 4980 MRSA isolates obtained between 1995 and 2004 found that the proportion of MRSA with high-level mupirocin resistance increased from 1.6% in the first 5 years of surveillance (1995–1999) to 7.0% in 2000 to 2004 ($P < .001$).

Community-acquired MRSA (CA-MRSA) isolates were more likely to show high-level resistance ($P = .05$). Patients who had resistant strains were more likely to be colonized with MRSA ($P = .04$), and the resistant strains were also more likely to be resistant to fusidic acid ($P < .001$). Evidence was seen of plasmid transmission and clonal spread.[24]

A study of surgical ICU patients showed that 13.2% of 302 MRSA isolates were resistant to mupirocin, with an 8.6% incidence of high-level resistance. Patients who had mupirocin-resistant MRSA were more likely to die in the hospital ($P = .027$). The isolates were predominately health care–type strains.[25]

ALTERNATIVES TO MUPIROCIN

Little evidence shows resistance to triple antibiotic ointment containing neomycin, polymyxin B, and bacitracin in Australia, where it has remained a prescription drug, or in the United States, where it has been available over-the-counter since the 1970s. Despite decades of use, both mupirocin-resistant S aureus and coagulase-negative staphylococci remain susceptible.[26] Bacitracin, polymyxin B, and gramicidin ointment eradicated MRSA colonization in 9 of 11 patients (82%), 10 of whom had undergone a 1-week course of topical mupirocin that failed. Mupirocin resistance was documented in 5 of the patients.[27]

Topical silver sulfadiazine can also treat MRSA infections effectively.[28] Silver sulphadiazine shows antistaphylococcal activity at concentrations of 64 µg/mL and retains activity against mupirocin-resistant strains. Commercial preparations contain much higher doses (10 mg/g), an therefore inhibitory concentrations should be achievable in tissue. Silver sulphadiazine shows promise for nasal decolonization, especially when used together with cerium nitrate.[29]

NEW TOPICAL ANTIBIOTICS

Retapamulin, a pleuromutilin marketed as a topical antibacterial for treating skin infections, is effective against staphylococci, including MRSA. It also shows activity against gram-negative bacteria, including 71% of *Bacteroides fragilis*. Based on inhibitory concentrations, it is more active than clindamycin and metronidazole against *Propionibacterium acnes* and anaerobic gram-positive cocci.[30] In vitro MIC(90)s of retapamulin against *S aureus* and *Streptococcus pyogenes* have been measured at 0.12 µg/mL and 0.016 µg/mL, respectively. Retapamulin also shows an in vitro postantibiotic residual effect, suggesting that success may be achieved even when compliance is less than perfect.[31]

Topical indolmycin demonstrates good antistaphylococcal activity and seems promising for treating MRSA strains resistant to fusidic acid and mupirocin. The agent is bacteriostatic but shows good in vitro activity against MSSA, MRSA, and vancomycin-intermediate *S aureus* (VISA), including strains resistant to mupirocin and fusidic acid. Some indolmycin-resistant strains have emerged, with high-level resistance most commonly associated with an H43N mutation in tryptophanyl-tRNA synthetase, the target enzyme of indolmycin.[32]

Nadifloxacin, a broad-spectrum quinolone, is approved for topical treatment of acne vulgaris and skin infections in Japan. One isomer shows promise as a systemic agent against MRSA, which has prompted some experts to suggest that nadifloxacin should be reserved for this use rather than risking widespread resistance through topical use. Others have advocated restricting its use as short-term treatment of skin infections but not chronic acne therapy.[33]

Rifalazil and other benzoxazinorifamycins are modified rifamycins that contain a distinct planar benzoxazine ring. Rifalazil shows high tissue penetration and achieves high intracellular levels. Drugs within this family are promising as topical agents, but resistance has been a significant problem with rifampin, and the potential for development of resistance to topical forms deserves careful scrutiny.[34]

ALTERNATIVES TO ANTIBIOTICS

As antibiotic resistance continues to emerge, alternatives need to be sought for the topical treatment of skin disorders. Honey and sugar are ancient remedies for chronic ulcers. More recently, the topical application of a paste of 70% sugar and 3% povidone-iodine was shown to accelerate healing in a diabetic mouse model of MRSA-infected ulcers. The paste significantly accelerated reepithelialization ($P < .01$) and decreased colony-forming units ($P < .05$).[35] The effect of the sugar is largely mediated by hypertonicity, and resistance is unlikely to develop.

Antibiotic products typically contain a single agent with a single mechanism of action. In contrast, botanicals contain thousands of synergistic components. Although the exact mechanisms of action are generally unknown, botanical agents have been used for centuries for the topical treatment of skin disease. The safety and efficacy of most of these agents have not been evaluated systematically, but some peer-reviewed data exist. Topical application of components of eucalyptus oil has been reported to show clinical activity in the setting of MRSA skin infections.[36] Essential oils from the stem, leaves, and fruits of Jamaican *Bursera simaruba* (Red Birch) and *Bursera lunanii* (Black Birch) show antibacterial activity against MRSA and MSSA, beta-hemolytic streptococci, *Escherichia coli*, *Proteus mirabilis*, and *Pseudomonas aeruginosa*.[37] For the eradication of MRSA colonization, a combination of a 4% tea tree oil nasal ointment and 5% tea tree oil body wash compared favorably with combination of 2% mupirocin nasal ointment and triclosan body wash.[38] Although these data should be regarded as preliminary, they suggest that further study of botanical agents is justified.

Topical gentian violet is messy and tastes terrible, but has been used for decades to treat oral thrush and skin infections. Topical gentian violet shows activity against MRSA. Minimum inhibitory concentration (MIC) for sensitive strains was 0.03 µg/mL. Similar to chlorhexidine, patients who have a perforated ear drum have the potential to develop middle ear toxicity.[39] In one study, gentian violet was used to eradicate colonization, but applications had to be continued for longer than 1 week.[40] It is unlikely that many patients would tolerate the mess and inconvenience.

Topical silver products are widely promoted in the wound care arena. Nanocrystalline technology improves the delivery of silver to a wound. Although randomized controlled trials are needed to prove efficacy, clinical experience has been good, with little evidence of toxicity.[41] In a comparison of a silver-coated dressing (Acticoat), chlorhexidine acetate 0.5% (Bactigrass), and fusidic acid 2% (Fucidin) in MRSA-contaminated, full-skin thickness rat burn wounds, all treatments shows a clinical effect. However, the organism was recovered from the burn eschar of all groups except the fusidic acid group, which translated to superiority of fusidic acid for the major end points studied. Major end points did not differ significantly between the silver dressing and chlorhexidine acetate groups.[42]

Akacid plus is a promising new polymeric guanidine disinfectant that compares favorably with agents such as chlorhexidine digluconate and mupirocin. In vitro assays show good activity against S aureus. MIC90s of chlorhexidine and mupirocin can show 4- and 32-fold increases for MRSA compared with MSSA, whereas MICs with Akacid plus are similar for MRSA and MSSA.[43]

Group B streptococci (S agalactiae) causes substantial morbidity and mortality among newborns. Resistance is increasing to drugs such as erythromycin and clindamycin, which can be used in pregnant women allergic to penicillin. Topical agents such as benzalkonium chloride shows good MIC90 values against group B streptococci, including strains resistant to both erythromycin and clindamycin. This finding suggests that these agents may be useful in reducing vaginal group B streptococcus colonization in pregnant women before delivery.[44]

TOPICAL ANTIMICROBIALS ACTIVE AGAINST HIV

Various topical agents have been evaluated for activity against human immunodeficiency virus type 1 (HIV-1). In a study of the antiviral effects of various commercially available vaginal gels, cellular transfer of HIV-1 was inhibited by all products except Carraguard, KY-N9, and Vena Gel. Unfortunately, the agents that showed efficacy also had cellular cytotoxic effects.[45] The ultimate goal of topical agents that are well tolerated and have a good effect against the virus remains elusive.

RESISTANCE TO ANTIBIOTICS USED TO TREAT ACNE

As early as the 1970s, P acnes isolates began to show decreased sensitivity to some antibiotics commonly used to treat acne. The first clinically relevant changes in P acnes antibiotic sensitivity were noted in the United States shortly after the topical formulations of erythromycin and clindamycin were introduced. Strains with very high MIC levels for erythromycin and elevated MICs for tetracycline were reported by the late 1980s.[46] The use of oral erythromycin or topical clindamycin encourages the development of resistant propionibacteria, and resistant strains are associated with therapeutic failure.[47]

Emerging resistance has been a particular issue for erythromycin. A British review of 45 controlled trials noted a significant decrease in the effect of erythromycin on both inflammatory and noninflammatory lesion count over time (P = .001), whereas the efficacy of topical clindamycin remained stable during the study period.[48] Topical clindamycin currently retains better efficacy than topical erythromycin; however, the emergence and spread of resistance to both agents is of concern.[49]

Overuse of antibiotics may also contribute to the prevalence of other pathogens. In one study, 6 (10%) of 63 patients who were not using antibiotics had positive S pyogenes throat cultures compared with 13 (33%) of 42 patients using oral or topical antibiotics (P = .003). Of 13 isolates from those using antibiotics, 11 were resistant to tetracycline compared with 20% (1/5) of those not using antibiotics (P = .01).[50] Limitations of the study include the low numbers of patients in each study group and the lack of a clear mechanism for topical antibiotics predisposing to oropharyngeal carriage of an organism, but the study does raise concerns about appropriate antibiotic use.

Topical erythromycin is associated with a transient increased prevalence and density of resistant coagulase-negative staphylococci.[51] A study comparing resistance during use of erythromycin gel versus the vehicle alone found that the prevalence of erythromycin-resistant coagulase-negative Staphylococci on the face was already 87% at baseline, but increased to 98% by week 12 in the erythromycin-treated group. Resistant organisms were also noted on the untreated back and in the nares.[52] Benzoyl peroxide added to erythromycin prevents the emergence of erythromycin-resistant coagulase-negative staphylococci.[53]

Skin cultures from 622 European patients who had acne showed that the prevalence of isolates resistant to at least one antibiotic was lowest in Hungary (51%) and highest in Spain (94%). Resistance patterns were strongly correlated with prescribing habits. Combined resistance to clindamycin and erythromycin was noted in 91% of isolates in Spain and was far more common overall than resistance to the tetracyclines, which was highest in the United Kingdom (26.4%). Resistant propionibacteria were common on the skin of untreated contacts, suggesting that widespread use of topical antibiotics promotes the spread of resistant organisms within the community.[54]

STRATEGIES TO REDUCE EMERGENCE OF RESISTANCE

The primary strategy to stem the emergence of resistance to topical antibiotics is the concurrent use of benzoyl peroxide. A study of clindamycin phosphate 1%/benzoyl peroxide 5% gel versus clindamycin 1% gel found that clindamycin-resistant P acnes count was significantly reduced after 16 weeks of treatment with combination gel versus clindamycin monotherapy (P = .018).[55]

Another alternative is to manage acne with non-antibiotic topicals, such as retinoids, azalaic acid, or topical antiandrogens. Although retinoids are typically used in acne regimens, no evidence shows that they prevent antibiotic resistance when used in combination with a topical antibiotic. Even when the therapeutic response is inadequate for initial therapy, nonantibiotic topicals are attractive for maintenance to limit exposure to antibiotics. A double-blind, randomized, placebo-controlled study in 33 patients suggested that a combination of triethyl citrate or ethyl linoleate can be effective against inflammatory and noninflammatory lesions.[56] Topical nicotinamide also shows some promise in the treatment of acne. Preliminary data suggest that 4% nicotinamide has comparable efficacy to 1% clindamycin in treating acne vulgaris.[57]

New antibiotics are being studied, including new topical macrolides. BAL19403, which belongs to a new family of macrolide antibiotics, shows excellent in vitro activity against propionibacteria, including erythromycin- and clindamycin-resistant propionibacteria.[58] A double-blind study comparing nadifloxacin 1% cream with erythromycin 2% cream for the treatment of mild-to-moderate acne vulgaris showed similar reduction of P acnes and efficacy between the groups.[59]

Zinc compounds deserve further study as topical agents for the treatment of acne. Zinc salts have an anti-inflammatory effect and bacteriostatic activity against P acnes and Micrococcaceae, including erythromycin-resistant species.[60]

A small randomized, single-blind study compared topical clindamycin/benzoyl peroxide to erythromycin/zinc acetate for the treatment of mild to moderate facial acne vulgaris. Both treatments were well tolerated, but clindamcyin/benzoyl peroxide showed an earlier onset of action.[61] Oral zinc gluconate, 30 mg, daily for 2 months results in a reduction in the number of inflammatory acne lesions. Zinc shows some promise as an agent to stem the emergence of resistant bacteria. Addition of zinc salts to the culture media reduced resistance of P acnes strains to erythromycin in vitro.[62] These preliminary data must be validated through clinical trials.

Botanical compounds also deserve study in the setting of acne vulgaris. A study of various botanical extracts for antimicrobial activity against 29 aerobic and anaerobic bacteria and yeasts showed that Usnea barbata and its major component usnic acid were the most active compounds, especially in anaerobic bacteria. Usnea extract also inhibited several gram-positive species, including MRSA strains. Activity was present against P acnes, Corynebacterium spp, and Malassezia furfur. Rosmarinus, Salvia, Boswellia, and Harpagophytum extracts also had antibacterial activity.[63]

SUMMARY

Emerging resistance to topical antimicrobials is of concern. Responsible use of antibiotics includes using them only when a clear medical indication exists, using them only as long as necessary to achieve the desired effect, using combination therapy that minimizes the emergence of resistance, and using alternatives to antibiotics when possible.

REFERENCES

1. Desrosiers M, Bendouah Z, Barbeau J. Effectiveness of topical antibiotics on Staphylococcus aureus biofilm in vitro. Am J Rhinol 2007;21(2):149–53.
2. Dohmen PM. Influence of skin flora and preventive measures on surgical site infection during cardiac surgery. Surg Infect (Larchmt) 2006;7(Suppl 1): S13–7.
3. Smack DP, Harrington AC, Dunn C, et al. Infection and allergy incidence in ambulatory surgery patients using white petrolatum vs bacitracin ointment. A randomized controlled trial. JAMA 1996;276(12):972–7.
4. Rahimian J, Khan R, LaScalea KA. Does nasal colonization or mupirocin treatment affect recurrence of methicillin-resistant Staphylococcus aureus skin and skin structure infections? Infect Control Hosp Epidemiol 2007;28(12):1415–6.
5. Wendt C, Schinke S, Württemberger M, et al. Value of whole-body washing with chlorhexidine for the eradication of methicillin-resistant Staphylococcus aureus: a randomized, placebo-controlled, double-blind clinical trial. Infect Control Hosp Epidemiol 2007;28(9):1036–43.
6. Fawley WN, Parnell P, Hall J, et al. Surveillance for mupirocin resistance following introduction of routine peri-operative prophylaxis with nasal mupirocin. J Hosp Infect 2006;62(3):327–32.
7. Gould IM, MacKenzie FM, MacLennan G, et al. Topical antimicrobials in combination with admission screening and barrier precautions to control endemic methicillin-resistant Staphylococcus aureus in an intensive care unit. Int J Antimicrob Agents 2007;29(5):536–43.
8. Simor AE, Phillips E, McGeer A, et al. Randomized controlled trial of chlorhexidine gluconate for washing, intranasal mupirocin, and rifampin and doxycycline versus no treatment for the eradication of methicillin-resistant Staphylococcus aureus colonization. Clin Infect Dis 2007;44(2):178–85.

9. Kniehl E, Becker A, Forster DH. Bed, bath and beyond: pitfalls in prompt eradication of methicillin-resistant Staphylococcus aureus carrier status in healthcare workers. J Hosp Infect 2005;59(3):180–7.

10. Kanazawa K, Ueda Y. Bactericial activity of chlorhexidine gluconate against recent clinical isolates of various bacterial species in Japan. Jpn J Antibiot 2004;57(5):449–64.

11. Zhang YH, Liu XY, Zhu LL, et al. Study on the resistance of methicillin-resistant staphylococcus aureus to iodophor and chlorhexidine. Zhonghua Liu Xing Bing Xue Za Zhi 2004;25(3):248–50.

12. Kampf G, Jarosch R, Ruden H. Limited effectiveness of chlorhexidine based hand disinfectants against methicillin-resistant Staphylococcus aureus (MRSA). J Hosp Infect 1998;38(4):297–303.

13. Suzuki J, Komatsuzawa H, Kozai K, et al. In vitro susceptibility of Staphylococcus aureus including MRSA to four disinfectants. ASDC J Dent Child 1997;64(4):260–3.

14. Block C, Robenshtok E, Simhon A, et al. Evaluation of chlorhexidine and povidone iodine activity against methicillin-resistant Staphylococcus aureus and vancomycin-resistant Enterococcus faecalis using a surface test. J Hosp Infect 2000;46(2):147–52.

15. Suller MT, Russell AD. Antibiotic and biocide resistance in methicillin-resistant Staphylococcus aureus and vancomycin-resistant enterococcus. J Hosp Infect 1999;43(4):281–91.

16. Brenwald NP, Fraise AP. Triclosan resistance in methicillin-resistant Staphylococcus aureus (MRSA). J Hosp Infect 2003;55(2):141–4.

17. Bamber AI, Neal TJ. An assessment of triclosan susceptibility in methicillin-resistant and methicillin-sensitive Staphylococcus aureus. J Hosp Infect 1999; 41(2):107–9.

18. Lambert RJ. Comparative analysis of antibiotic and antimicrobial biocide susceptibility data in clinical isolates of methicillin-sensitive Staphylococcus aureus, methicillin-resistant Staphylococcus aureus and Pseudomonas aeruginosa between 1989 and 2000. J Appl Microbiol 2004;97(4):699–711.

19. Noguchi N, Suwa J, Narui K, et al. Susceptibilities to antiseptic agents and distribution of antiseptic-resistance genes qacA/B and smr of methicillin-resistant Staphylococcus aureus isolated in Asia during 1998 and 1999. J Med Microbiol 2005;54(Pt 6):557–65.

20. Suller MT, Russell AD. Triclosan and antibiotic resistance in Staphylococcus aureus. J Antimicrob Chemother 2000;46(1):11–8.

21. Acikel C, Oncul O, Ulkur E, et al. Comparison of silver sulfadiazine 1%, mupirocin 2%, and fusidic acid 2% for topical antibacterial effect in methicillin-resistant staphylococci-infected, full-skin thickness rat burn wounds. J Burn Care Rehabil 2003;24(1):37–41.

22. Afset JE, Maeland JA. Streptococcus pyogenes to topical antibiotics: indications of clonal spread of fusidic acid-resistant Staphylococcus aureus. Scand J Infect Dis 2003;35(2):84–9.

23. Mulvey MR, MacDougall L, Cholin B, Saskatchewan CA-MRSA Study Group, et al. Community-associated methicillin-resistant Staphylococcus aureus, Canada. Emerg Infect Dis 2005;11(6):844–50.

24. Simor AE, Stuart TL, Louie L, et al. Canadian Nosocomial Infection Surveillance Program (CNISP). Mupirocin-Resistant, Methicillin-Resistant Staphylococcus aureus (MRSA) in Canadian Hospitals. Antimicrob Agents Chemother 2007;. [Epub ahead of print].

25. Jones JC, Rogers TJ, Brookmeyer P, et al. Mupirocin resistance in patients colonized with methicillin-resistant Staphylococcus aureus in a surgical intensive care unit. Clin Infect Dis 2007;45(5):541–7.

26. Jones RN, Li Q, Kohut B, et al. Contemporary antimicrobial activity of triple antibiotic ointment: a multiphased study of recent clinical isolates in the United States and Australia. Diagn Microbiol Infect Dis 2006;54(1):63–71.

27. Fung S, O'Grady S, Kennedy C, et al. The utility of polysporin ointment in the eradication of methicillin-resistant Staphylococcus aureus colonization: a pilot study. Infect Control Hosp Epidemiol 2000; 21(10):653–5.

28. Tehrani R. Silver sulphadiazine for MRSA infections. Indian J Dermatol Venereol Leprol 2004;70(3):186.

29. Schuenck RP, Dadalti P, Silva MG, et al. Oxacillin- and mupirocin-resistant Staphylococcus aureus: in vitro activity of silver sulphadiazine and cerium nitrate in hospital strains. J Chemother 2004;16(5):453–8.

30. Odou MF, Muller C, Calvet L, et al. In vitro activity against anaerobes of retapamulin, a new topical antibiotic for treatment of skin infections. J Antimicrob Chemother 2007;59(4):646–51.

31. Rittenhouse S, Biswas S, Broskey J, et al. Selection of retapamulin, a novel pleuromutilin for topical use. Antimicrob Agents Chemother 2006;50(11):3882–5.

32. Hurdle JG, O'Neill AJ, Chopra I. Anti-staphylococcal activity of indolmycin, a potential topical agent for control of staphylococcal infections. J Antimicrob Chemother 2004;54(2):549–52.

33. Jacobs MR, Appelbaum PC. Nadifloxacin: a quinolone for topical treatment of skin infections and potential for systemic use of its active isomer, WCK 771. Expert Opin Pharmacother 2006;7(14):1957–66.

34. Rothstein DM, Shalish C, Murphy CK, et al. Development potential of rifalazil and other benzoxazinorifamycins. Expert Opin Investig Drugs 2006;15(6):603–23.

35. Shi CM, Nakao H, Yamazaki M, et al. Mixture of sugar and povidone-iodine stimulates healing of MRSA-infected skin ulcers on db/db mice. Arch Dermatol Res 2007; [Epub ahead of print].

36. Sherry E, Boeck H, Warnke PH. Topical application of a new formulation of eucalyptus oil phytochemical

clears methicillin-resistant Staphylococcus aureus infection. Am J Infect Control 2001;29(5):346.

37. Junor GO, Porter RB, Facey PC, et al. Investigation of essential oil extracts from four native Jamaican species of Bursera for antibacterial activity. West Indian Med J 2007;56(1):22–5.

38. Caelli M, Porteous J, Carson CF, et al. Tea tree oil as an alternative topical decolonization agent for methicillin-resistant Staphylococcus aureus. J Hosp Infect 2000;46(3):236–7.

39. Kayama C, Goto Y, Shimoya S, et al. Effects of gentian violet on refractory discharging ears infected with methicillin-resistant Staphylococcus aureus. J Otolaryngol 2006;35(6):384–6.

40. Okano M, Noguchi S, Tabata K, et al. Topical gentian violet for cutaneous infection and nasal carriage with MRSA. Int J Dermatol 2000;39(12):942–4.

41. Leaper DJ. Silver dressings: their role in wound management. Int Wound J 2006;3(4):282–94.

42. Ulkür E, Oncul O, Karagoz H, et al. Comparison of silver-coated dressing (Acticoat), chlorhexidine acetate 0.5% (Bactigrass), and fusidic acid 2% (Fucidin) for topical antibacterial effect in methicillin-resistant Staphylococci-contaminated, full-skin thickness rat burn wounds. Burns 2005;31(7):874–7.

43. Buxbaum A, Kratzer C, Graninger W, et al. Antimicrobial and toxicological profile of the new biocide Akacid plus. J Antimicrob Chemother 2006;58(1):193–7.

44. Mosca A, Russo F, Miragliotta G. In vitro antimicrobial activity of benzalkonium chloride against clinical isolates of Streptococcus agalactiae. J Antimicrob Chemother 2006;57(3):566–8.

45. Dezzutti CS, James VN, Ramos A, et al. In vitro comparison of topical microbicides for prevention of human immunodeficiency virus type 1 transmission. Antimicrob Agents Chemother 2004;48(10):3834–44.

46. Eady EA, Gloor M, Leyden JJ. Propionibacterium acnes resistance: a worldwide problem. Dermatology 2003;206(1):54–6.

47. Eady EA, Cove JH, Holland KT, et al. Erythromycin resistant propionibacteria in antibiotic treated acne patients: association with therapeutic failure. Br J Dermatol 1989;121(1):51–7.

48. Simonart T, Dramaix M. Treatment of acne with topical antibiotics: lessons from clinical studies. Br J Dermatol 2005;153(2):395–403.

49. Guay DR. Topical clindamycin in the management of acne vulgaris. Expert Opin Pharmacother 2007;8(15):2625–64.

50. Levy RM, Huang EY, Roling D, et al. Effect of antibiotics on the oropharyngeal flora in patients with acne. Arch Dermatol 2003;139(4):467–71.

51. Vowels BR, Feingold DS, Sloughfy C, et al. Effects of topical erythromycin on ecology of aerobic cutaneous bacterial flora. Antimicrob Agents Chemother 1996;40(11):2598–604.

52. Mills O Jr, Thornsberry C, Cardin CW, et al. Bacterial resistance and therapeutic outcome following three months of topical acne therapy with 2% erythromycin gel versus its vehicle. Acta Derm Venereol 2002;82(4):260–5.

53. Harkaway KS, McGinley KJ, Foglia AN, et al. Antibiotic resistance patterns in coagulase-negative staphylococci after treatment with topical erythromycin, benzoyl peroxide, and combination therapy. Br J Dermatol 1992;126(6):586–90.

54. Ross JI, Snelling AM, Carnegie E, et al. Antibiotic-resistant acne: lessons from Europe. Br J Dermatol 2003;148(3):467–78.

55. Cunliffe WJ, Holland KT, Bojar R, et al. A randomized, double-blind comparison of a clindamycin phosphate/benzoyl peroxide gel formulation and a matching clindamycin gel with respect to microbiologic activity and clinical efficacy in the topical treatment of acne vulgaris. Clin Ther 2002;24(7):1117–33.

56. Charakida A, Charakida M, Chu AC. Double-blind, randomized, placebo-controlled study of a lotion containing triethyl citrate and ethyl linoleate in the treatment of acne vulgaris. Br J Dermatol 2007;157(3):569–74.

57. Shalita AR, Smith JG, Parish LC, et al. Topical nicotinamide compared with clindamycin gel in the treatment of inflammatory acne vulgaris. Int J Dermatol 1995;34(6):434–7.

58. Heller S, Kellenberger L, Shapiro S. Antipropionibacterial activity of BAL19403, a novel macrolide antibiotic. Antimicrob Agents Chemother 2007;51(6):1956–61.

59. Plewig G, Holland KT, Nenoff P. Clinical and bacteriological evaluation of nadifloxacin 1% cream in patients with acne vulgaris: a double-blind, phase III comparison study versus erythromycin 2% cream. Eur J Dermatol 2006;16(1):48–55.

60. Fluhr JW, Bösch B, Gloor M, et al. In-vitro and in-vivo efficacy of zinc acetate against propionibacteria alone and in combination with erythromycin. Zentralbl Bakteriol 1999;289(4):445–56.

61. Langner A, Sheehan-Dare R, Layton A. A randomized, single-blind comparison of topical clindamycin + benzoyl peroxide (Duac) and erythromycin + zinc acetate (Zineryt) in the treatment of mild to moderate facial acne vulgaris. J Eur Acad Dermatol Venereol 2007;21(3):311–9.

62. Dreno B, Foulc P, Reynaud A, et al. Effect of zinc gluconate on propionibacterium acnes resistance to erythromycin in patients with inflammatory acne: in vitro and in vivo study. Eur J Dermatol 2005;15(3):152–5.

63. Weckesser S, Engel K, Simon-Haarhaus B, et al. Screening of plant extracts for antimicrobial activity against bacteria and yeasts with dermatological relevance. Phytomedicine 2007;14(7–8):508–16.

Optimizing Use of Oral Antibiotics in Acne Vulgaris

James Q. Del Rosso, DO, FAOCD*, Grace Kim, DO

KEYWORDS

• Oral antibiotics • Acne vulgaris • Antibiotic resistance

Several suggestions have been published on optimal use of oral antibiotics for treating acne vulgaris, directed at achieving optimal therapeutic results while reducing the potential for antibiotic resistance. Examples include limiting the duration of therapy, using combination therapy regimens with a rational topical program from the outset, avoiding unnecessary switching of oral antibiotics, and incorporating a benzoyl peroxide–containing formulation to reduce emergence of antibiotic-resistant Propionibacterium acnes strains. Potential adverse reactions and drug interactions associated with specific oral antibiotics are also important considerations.

Acne vulgaris is the most common disorder encountered in dermatology practice, accounting for 3.8 million office visits, or 11.3% of total visits to non-Federal office–based dermatologists in the United States in 2004.[1] Most patients are teenagers, accounting for more than 2 million visits per year for managing acne vulgaris.[2] Prepubertal onset is not uncommon, and many patients experience acne beyond teenage years, with 10% of visits reported to occur between ages 35 and 44 years.[2,3] Acne vulgaris is well established as a disease state associated with a significant psychosocial burden, negatively impacting quality of life of many affected patients.[4,5]

PATHOPHYSIOLOGY OF ACNE VULGARIS

Although the pathogenesis of acne vulgaris is multifactorial, a commensal skin bacterium, P acnes, is believed to play a major role in the formation of inflammatory acne lesions, and possibly comedogenesis.[6–8] P acnes has been shown to trigger innate immune response and the inflammatory cascade in acne vulgaris through interacting with toll-like receptors (TLRs) in the skin, specifically TLR-2, which are expressed on inflammatory cells such as monocytes, macrophages, neutrophils, dendritic cells, and keratinocytes.[9,10] Available data based on more recent analysis of the P acnes genome, research evaluating inflammation and comedogenesis in acne vulgaris, microbiologic studies evaluating P acnes reduction performed in vivo and in vitro, and results observed in clinical trials support suppressing P acnes with antimicrobial therapy as part of the management plan in patients who have acne vulgaris.[6–12] Additionally, some antibiotics, especially tetracycline derivatives, exhibit anti-inflammatory effects unrelated to their antibiotic properties, which are believed to contribute to their therapeutic benefit in inflammatory skin disorders, including acne vulgaris.[11,13,14]

USE OF ORAL ANTIBIOTICS IN ACNE MANAGEMENT

Usage data based on prescribing patterns from 2001 to 2006 in the United States show that dermatologists in office-based practice prescribe 8 to 9 million oral antibiotic prescriptions per year; two thirds of dermatologist prescriptions comprised tetracycline derivatives, primarily minocycline and doxycycline.[15,16] Most oral antibiotics prescribed by dermatologists were for treating acne vulgaris and rosacea. The number of topical antibiotics prescribed by dermatologists primarily for acne vulgaris in the United States from 2001 to 2006 was 3 to 4 million per year.[15,16]

Valley Hospital Medical Center, 620 Shadow Lane, Las Vegas, NV 89106, USA
* Corresponding author. 880 Seven Hills Drive, Suite 260, Henderson, NV 89052.
E-mail address: jqdelrosso@yahoo.com (J.Q. Del Rosso).

Dermatol Clin 27 (2009) 33–42
doi:10.1016/j.det.2008.07.006

derm.theclinics.com

Until the extended-release tablet formulation of minocycline was approved in 2006 by the U.S. Food and Drug Administration (FDA), oral antibiotics were used in the United States for acne vulgaris based solely on clinical experience and a relatively sparse collection of clinical studies, and without FDA approval from pivotal phase III clinical trials.[17–19]

The main oral antibiotics used for treating acne vulgaris included tetracycline, minocycline, doxycycline, and erythromycin.[2,11,19–22] More recently in the United States, minocycline and doxycycline are used more frequently than tetracycline and erythromycin because of increased resistance of P acnes to the latter two agents.[11] However, a trend has gradually emerged toward an increase in P acnes organisms becoming less sensitive to doxycycline and minocycline, correlating with their extent of use.[11,23–25]

Oral tetracycline and oxytetracycline have been available since the mid-1950s, doxycycline since 1967, and minocycline since 1972.[13] Two reviews of clinical studies of acne vulgaris evaluating tetracycline, doxycycline, and immediate-release minocycline found 12 studies, involving 953 patients, completed between 1969 and 2001.[19–21] The efficacy and safety profile of extended-release minocycline tablets included evaluation of weight-based dosing and was determined before FDA approval based on a phase II dose-finding study and two phase III pivotal trials collectively inclusive of 1038 subjects.[18] Other alternative oral antibiotics reported to be useful for treating acne vulgaris include trimethoprim/sulfamethoxazole and azithromycin.[26–28]

RATIONALE FOR ORAL ANTIBIOTIC USE IN ACNE VULGARIS

The use of oral antibiotics, especially tetracyclines and erythromycin, has been based primarily on clinical experience and observation followed subsequently by intermittently performed clinical studies.[17–19] The use of extended-release minocycline tablets, prescribed at a dosage of 1 mg/kg once daily is based on data from large-scale pivotal trials and FDA approval in the United States.[17,18] Data on log reduction in P acnes organism counts after treatment with individual antibiotics have been summarized elsewhere. Among the most commonly prescribed oral antibiotics for acne vulgaris, the greatest reduction in P acnes has been documented with minocycline, followed in order by doxycycline, tetracycline, and erythromycin.[29]

The clinical efficacy of oral antibiotics in the treatment of acne vulgaris, and recommendations on their optimal use have been reported in the literature and are reviewed elsewhere.[2,11,12,17–22]

INDICATIONS FOR ORAL ANTIBIOTIC USE IN ACNE VULGARIS

The primary indication for oral antibiotic therapy in acne vulgaris is moderate to severe inflammatory involvement on the face or trunk.[12] **Table 1** depicts the dosing schedule of oral antibiotics commonly used for treating acne vulgaris.

ROLE OF COMBINATION THERAPY WHEN PRESCRIBING AN ORAL ANTIBIOTIC FOR ACNE VULGARIS

Antibiotic monotherapy should be avoided because of promotion of antibiotic resistance; oral antibiotic therapy is best used in combination with a topical regimen that includes a benzoyl peroxide–containing formulation and a topical retinoid.[11,12,30,31] Combination therapy using a rational topical regimen along with an oral antibiotic is an optimal approach in patients who have moderate to severe acne vulgaris.[11,30]

Experts have recommended that benzoyl peroxide therapy be initiated if antibiotic treatment is used for more than 2 months.[12] However, including a benzoyl peroxide–containing formulation as part of the overall combination therapy regimen from the outset seems more rational, because this agent by itself is effective in reducing inflammatory acne lesions and moderately reduces noninflammatory acne lesions.[12,32,33] In addition, benzoyl peroxide has been shown to reduce the emergence of antibiotic-resistant strains of P acnes and to suppress preexisting P acnes organisms resistant to multiple antibiotics, including erythromycin, tetracycline, doxycycline, and minocycline.[11,29–31,34,35]

Another recommendation suggests that concomitant use of oral and topical antibiotics that are chemically dissimilar be avoided because of concern about development of multidrug-resistant bacterial strains.[12,36] The authors find no definitive scientific support for this recommendation in the literature. This recommendation seems to be rational and scientifically based in the absence of benzoyl peroxide use; however, concomitant use of benzoyl peroxide would be expected to counteract emergence of P acnes resistance. Experts have also suggested that a short course of benzoyl peroxide therapy (eg, 2 to 3 weeks) be used before initiation of antibiotic therapy to help eradicate antibiotic-resistant P acnes strains, an approach that may improve the overall efficacy of antibiotic treatment.[12,35–37]

Table 1
Oral antibiotic agents commonly used for treatment of acne vulgaris

Drug	Usual Dosage Range	Comments	Refs
Minocycline (immediate-release)	50–100 mg once or twice daily	Vestibular reactions seem to be dose-related and more common with immediate-release formulations (especially generic)	11,19–22,26
Minocycline (extended-release)	1 mg/kg per day (45–135 mg once daily)	Efficacy comparable to 2 mg/kg per day and 3 mg/kg per day; potential for vestibular reactions lower than with immediate release formulations	17,18
Doxycycline	75–100 mg once or twice daily 150 mg once daily	Photosensitivity reported to be dose-related (higher potential at ≥ 100 mg/d)	19–22,26
Trimethoprim/ Sulfamethoxazole	160 mg/800 mg trimethoprim+sulfamethoxazole once or twice daily	Used in cases refractory to other oral antibiotics or for gram-negative acne; trimethoprim alone reported at dose of 300 mg twice daily	22,26,27

Data from Refs.[11,19,21,22].

CONCERN ABOUT ORAL ANTIBIOTIC THERAPY IN ACNE VULGARIS AND DEVELOPMENT OF ANTIBIOTIC RESISTANCE

Changing patterns in antibiotic resistance that develop over time because of selection pressure and transfer of antibiotic resistance genes have led to the emergence of organisms less sensitive to previously effective antibiotics, which are of specific interest to dermatologists.[38] These include erythromycin- and tetracycline-resistant *P acnes*, macrolide-resistant pathogenic streptococci and staphylococci, mupirocin-resistant *Staphylococcus aureus*, and community-acquired methicillin-resistant *S aureus* (CA-MRSA).[11,15,38]

As long ago as 1983, long-term oral antibiotic therapy administered over a mean duration of 21 months was associated with an increase in minimum inhibitory concentration (MIC) for *P acnes* of up to 5-fold for tetracycline and 100-fold for erythromycin compared with acne-free control subjects and those not receiving antibiotics.[39] Additional reports have addressed the concern about emergence of *P acnes* strains less sensitive to multiple antibiotics used to treat acne vulgaris, including topical and oral agents.[23–25,36,40–43] Data collected from studies completed in the United Kingdom support the observation of an increasing trend in resistance of *P acnes* to erythromycin, clindamycin, or tetracycline, observed to be 20% in 1988, 38 % in 1993, 49% in 1995, and 62% in 1996.[43]

In the United States, although a slight trend toward decreased prescribing of oral antibiotics by dermatologists has been suggested based on annual reviews of prescribing patterns, the trend has been flat with only a modest overall decline from 2001 to 2006.[15,16] An analysis of trends in prescribing of acne medications in the United States from the 1990–2002 National Ambulatory Medical Care Survey reported a marked decline in the use of several drug classes that depend on antimicrobial activity, such as benzoyl peroxide, topical clindamycin, oral erythromycin, and oral tetracycline agents, with an increase in nonantimicrobial therapies, such as topical retinoids and oral isotretinoin.[44] The launch in the United States in 1996 of an FDA-mandated safety registry (iPledge program) for all clinicians who prescribe oral iso-tretinoin and for all patients treated with the drug has resulted in a decrease in the number of isotretinoin prescriptions, a factor which is likely to result in continued and increased dependence on oral antibiotic therapy for acne vulgaris, including chronic use.

Because of concerns in the United Kingdom about antibiotic resistance, initiatives to modify how antibiotics are prescribed for acne vulgaris emerged in the early 1990s with continued emphasis into the millennium.[38–40] From 1995 to 2000, antibiotic prescriptions for acne declined by 33% in the United Kingdom, with most of the decline comprising oral antibiotic agents; topical antibiotic prescriptions declined by 12% over that same period.[25,45]

EFFECTS OF *PROPIONIBACTERIUM ACNES* ANTIBIOTIC RESISTANCE ON RESPONSE TO ANTIBIOTIC THERAPY

In acne vulgaris, some studies have observed poor therapeutic response to antibiotics in patients who have microbiologically confirmed large quantities of *P acnes* that exhibit high MIC levels to macrolides and tetracyclines.[25,36,39,46] However, the correlation between prevalence of *P acnes* resistance and poor therapeutic response to antibiotic therapy is not always consistent.[11] Potential factors that may modify response to antibiotic therapy include preexisting antibiotic resistance, the quantity of antibiotic-resistant *P acnes* strains in the individual patient, resistance to multiple antibiotics, use of antibiotics without concomitant use of benzoyl peroxide, repeated courses of antibiotic therapy especially without concomitant use of benzoyl peroxide, unnecessary switching of oral antibiotic agents despite previous efficacy, individual antibiotic characteristics such as lipophilicity, and in vivo existence of *P acnes* in a protective extracellular polysaccharide biofilm.[11,12,17,18,22,36,39,47]

Despite documentation of widespread global prevalence of antibiotic-resistant *P acnes*, topical and oral antibiotics that have been used extensively over several years, such as topical clindamycin, oral minocycline, and oral doxycycline, continue to show efficacy in acne vulgaris.[11,18,48–51] Data from a pooled analysis of three recent 12-week trials completed with minocycline extended-release tablets in 1038 subjects who had moderate and severe acne vulgaris showed a mean percent reduction in inflammatory lesions of 45.5% in subjects treated with minocycline compared with 32.4% in those treated with placebo ($P<.001$).[51] Because these trials included

one phase II dose-ranging study and two pivotal phase III efficacy and safety studies, extended-release minocycline was used as monotherapy as mandated by protocols required to achieve FDA approval.[18] In the studies included in the pooled analysis, extended-release minocycline was dosed at 1 mg/kg administered once daily for 12 weeks.

In addition to their antibiotic activity that reduces *P acnes*, some antibiotics, including minocycline and doxycycline, may also improve acne vulgaris through direct anti-inflammatory mechanisms.[11,13,14,19,52]

ALTERNATIVE ORAL ANTIBIOTICS IN ACNE THERAPY

The major alternative oral antibiotics in the treatment of acne vulgaris are trimethoprim/sulfamethoxazole and azithromycin.[12,22–28] Oral trimethoprim alone has also been suggested as a third-line agent in acne treatment.[53] Trimethoprim/sulfamethoxazole has been reported to be effective in some patients who have acne vulgaris who become refractory to the conventionally used oral antibiotics over time.[26,27] Additionally, trimethoprim/sulfamethoxazole is often used to treat potentially serious cutaneous and systemic infections, such as those caused by CA-MRSA. As a result, its use in acne vulgaris is best reserved for selected cases because of the potential for antibiotic resistance.[27] Additionally, the low but possible risk for major side effects associated with trimethoprim/sulfamethoxazole are important considerations.[27]

Oral azithromycin has been reported to be effective in treating acne vulgaris in four open and two investigator-blinded clinical trials, inclusive of 187 subjects and 341 subjects, respectively, using various treatment regimens.[26,28] Most regimens with oral azithromycin have used intermittent dosing schedules, such as three 250 mg doses per week, because of a long terminal half-life of 68 hours.[26] Because azithromycin is commonly used to treat various systemic infections and intracellular pathogens, such *Chlamydia* spp and atypical *Mycobacterium* spp, its use in acne vulgaris is best reserved for selected cases to avoid the potential for development of resistant organisms.[26]

Oral cephalosporins and fluoroquinolones have also been sporadically reported to be effective for treating acne vulgaris.[26] However, because of the heavy dependence on fluoroquinolones and cephalosporins for treating various systemic and cutaneous infections, their use for treating acne vulgaris is discouraged overall. Exceptions may include short-term use for selected refractory cases and documented cases of gram-negative acne/folliculitis.

ROLE OF ORAL ANTIBIOTICS IN LONG-TERM THERAPY AND MAINTENANCE TREATMENT OF ACNE VULGARIS

Experts have suggested that oral antibiotic therapy for acne vulgaris, used in combination with a topical regimen comprising a retinoid and benzoyl peroxide–containing formulation, be administered over a minimum of 6 to 8 weeks and over a maximum of 12 weeks to 6 months.[11,12,22,30] At 6 to 8 weeks after therapy is initiated, clinicians may determine a substantial lack of efficacy and, if adequate compliance is assumed, a change in oral antibiotic therapy is reasonable.[22,47] However, if partial improvement is observed, continuing with the current regimen for an additional 6 to 8 weeks is reasonable to assess progress.

Once reasonable control of acne is observed to be stable, discontinuation of oral antibiotic therapy with continuation of the topical regimen is suggested usually over a period of 3 to 6 months.[12,22] Reasonable control may be defined as the observation of no new or a marked decrease in inflammatory lesions.[12] No consensus exists on whether oral antibiotic therapy should be discontinued abruptly or tapered.[11,12,22] Clinical judgment is warranted, with the authors favoring abrupt discontinuation of oral antibiotic therapy once new inflammatory lesions have significantly diminished or stopped and most residual inflammation secondary to resolving lesions has faded.

If repeated treatment with an oral antibiotic becomes necessary, experts suggest using the same oral antibiotic that was previously effective. The importance of benzoyl peroxide in suppressing less-sensitive *P acnes* organisms cannot be overemphasized.[11,12,22,34,35,45,47] Additionally, the role of topical retinoid therapy as a component of the initial and long-term maintenance regimen has been well established.[12,54]

Overall, the use of oral antibiotic therapy in the long-term management of acne vulgaris is not generally recommended.[12,22] However, individual patients may exhibit marked flares after discontinuing oral antibiotic therapy, despite the use of a rational topical maintenance program. Continuing the previously effective oral antibiotic in combination with the topical regimen may be necessary to sustain acceptable remission of acne lesions. In these cases, the problem may be inadequate compliance with the topical agents. Addressing the importance of adhering to treatment recommendations to successfully discontinue oral antibiotic therapy may be valuable.

Although data are limited, subantimicrobial therapy with doxycycline, using dosage regimens and formulations shown to exhibit anti-inflammatory activity without antibiotic effects, may be a "step down" option after discontinuing oral antibiotic therapy.[26,52] More studies are needed to better define the role of this therapeutic approach in the management of acne vulgaris.

OPTIMAL ADMINISTRATION OF ORAL ANTIBIOTICS

Some oral antibiotics are recommended to be administered with food to reduce the risk for gastrointestinal upset; however, this recommendation does not apply to all agents. Doxycycline, especially the hyclate salt, is best administered with food and a large glass of water to reduce gastrointestinal distress and esophagitis.[12,22] Doxycycline and minocycline may be administered with food; however, concomitant administration with iron supplements may decrease gastrointestinal absorption of both agents.[12,22] Reduced gastrointestinal absorption of the antibiotic may cause a diminished therapeutic response.

Although tetracycline is used less frequently than in the past, its absorption may be reduced and delayed with food. Concomitant ingestion of metal ions, such as calcium, magnesium, and aluminum found in many vitamin–mineral supplements and antacids, may also significantly reduce gastrointestinal absorption of tetracycline.[12,22] Although oral erythromycin is best administered with food to reduce gastrointestinal distress, azithromycin is recommended to be taken on an empty stomach because its absorption is diminished by food.[12,22,26] Unlike erythromycin, gastrointestinal upset is not commonly noted in patients treated with azithromycin.[26]

Agents that may cause gastrointestinal upset and esophagitis, such as erythromycin and doxycycline, should be ingested when the patient will be upright for at least a few hours, and not before anticipated reclining, such as before bedtime. An enteric-coated formulation of doxycycline reduces the potential for gastrointestinal upset and allows for once daily administration.

POTENTIAL ADVERSE REACTIONS OF ORAL ANTIBIOTICS USED FOR TREATING ACNE VULGARIS

All oral antibiotics used for treating acne vulgaris may be associated with nuisance side effects, such as gastrointestinal upset. The latter is most commonly observed with erythromycin and doxycycline.[12,22] Additionally, use of oral antibiotic therapy during pregnancy is not recommended.[12,22,26] Although it has been suggested that oral erythromycin is safe during pregnancy, these recommendations are not based on data evaluating chronic use over several months during pregnancy.[26]

Among the commonly prescribed oral antibiotics for acne vulgaris, doxycycline may result in dose-related phototoxicity.[12,19,22] Photoprotection education, including proper use of sunscreens or sunblocks affording protection against both ultraviolet (UV) A and UV-B, is recommended.

Minocycline has been associated with hyperpigmentation of skin and mucosa, including blue pigmentation of acne scars.[12,22] Although hyperpigmentation seems to be correlated with cumulative exposure to minocycline, the time course of onset and resolution is variable.[55] If hyperpigmentation is observed, discontinuing minocycline is recommended.

Although uncommon, drug hypersensitivity syndrome (DHS), characterized by fever, a diffuse exanthem-like skin eruption, and systemic abnormalities, including hepatitis and interstitial pneumonitis, has been reported with minocycline and trimethoprim/sulfamethoxazole.[56] DHS most commonly develops within 2 to 6 weeks after first exposure to the offending agent. Repeat exposure may cause onset of DHS within a few days. The most important component in the management of DHS is early recognition and discontinuation of the offending agent.

Although doxycycline and tetracycline have not been associated with development of DHS, absolute certainty about the absence of cross-reactivity between minocycline and other tetracycline derivatives is lacking.[56]

A lupus-like reaction has been reported in association with minocycline, most commonly in young women treated chronically over 1 to 2 years.[56] Characteristic findings include fever, malaise, and polyarthralgias. A cutaneous eruption is rarely noted, and may present as urticaria, vasculitis, or nonspecific erythema. Laboratory abnormalities may include elevated erythrocyte sedimentation rate, a positive antinuclear antibody test, significantly elevated hepatic enzymes, and a positivity for perinuclear antineutrophilic cytoplasmic antibodies directed against elastase or myeloperoxidase; positivity for antihistone antibodies is uncommon.[56] The lupus-like reaction associated with minocycline is reversible after discontinuation of the drug, although serologic positivity may persist for several months. Drug rechallenge is not recommended.

Trimethoprim/sulfamethoxazole may be associated with adverse reactions that are uncommon but potentially severe.[26,27] DHS associated with use of trimethoprim/sulfamethoxazole is discussed earlier. Severe cutaneous reactions, such as toxic epidermal necrolysis (TEN) and Stevens-Johnson syndrome (SJS) may occur, primarily within the first 1 to 2 months after initiation of therapy, and are associated with significant morbidity and mortality risks.[27] Hematologic reactions, including agranulocytosis, thrombocytopenia, and pancytopenia, have been reported with use of trimethoprim/sulfamethoxazole, but are fortunately uncommon.[27,57] The risk for hematologic toxicity associated with both short-term and long-term (≥ 3 months) use of trimethoprim/sulfamethoxazole seems to be increased in patients receiving higher than conventional doses, and in those who have preexisting folic acid deficiency or megaloblastic hematopoiesis characterized by elevated mean corpuscular volume or hypersegmented neutrophils.[57]

CLINICALLY SIGNIFICANT DRUG–DRUG INTERACTIONS ASSOCIATED WITH ORAL ANTIBIOTICS USED IN ACNE TREATMENT

Iron found in vitamin and mineral supplements may reduce gastrointestinal absorption of doxycycline and minocycline. Metal ions found in antacids, such as calcium, aluminum and magnesium, may reduce gastrointestinal absorption of tetracycline.[12,22]

Erythromycin may inhibit hepatic enzymes involved in the metabolism of other drugs, such as carbamazepine, cyclosporine, and some cholesterol lowering agents, such as lovastatin, simvastatin, and atorvastatin.[22] As a result, toxicity may result from significant elevations in serum level of the inhibited drug.

Trimethoprim/sulfamethoxazole should not be prescribed for patients on methotrexate because of an increased risk for serious hematologic reactions.[27,57]

FOLLOW-UP RECOMMENDATION FOR PATIENTS WHO HAVE ACNE TREATED WITH ORAL ANTIBIOTICS

Follow-up at 6 to 8 weeks is suggested to evaluate response to treatment, assess compliance, obtain patient feedback on ease of use and degree of satisfaction, evaluate tolerability and potential adverse effects, and determine whether to continue the current regimen or make changes. Unless a definite poor response, adverse reactions, or major compliance issues are noted, changing the treatment regimen without allowing an adequate duration of therapy to achieve a favorable therapeutic response leads to poor outcomes.

Major reasons to sustain periodic follow-up visits, such as every 6 to 12 weeks, include monitoring response, adjusting therapy, and encouraging continued compliance with treatment.[58] Periodic unsolicited phone calls from staff to address questions or concerns and enhance adherence with the treatment regimen have been suggested.[58] Prolonged intervals without professional follow-up and interaction frequently leads to decreased patient compliance.

Clinical assessment is the most important approach to monitoring for potential adverse reactions when an oral antibiotic is prescribed. When using agents associated with potentially serious adverse reactions, such as DHS, TEN or SJS, clinicians must inform patients to discontinue oral antibiotic therapy and contact the office if they experience a skin eruption or flu-like symptoms, such as fever, malaise, and sore throat. Although these symptoms may be unrelated to the oral antibiotic, they represent early signs of major adverse reactions, warranting a cautious approach. Clinicians may also chose to reevaluate the patient as early as 3 to 4 weeks.

No general recommendations exist for routinely performing baseline or periodic laboratory testing with oral antibiotics used to treat acne vulgaris. Experts have suggested that complete blood cell (CBC) testing with platelet count be performed at baseline and periodically in patients treated with trimethoprim/sulfamethoxazole.[57] As a general recommendation, no routine baseline or periodic laboratory monitoring is recommended in patients treated with tetracyclines, including minocycline.[56] Based on details related to the medical history of individual patients, clinicians may choose to avoid using a specific agent or to incorporate baseline or periodic laboratory monitoring.

CONCLUDING RECOMMENDATIONS

Oral antibiotics remain an important component of acne treatment, especially in patients who have moderate to severe disease affecting the face or trunk. Currently, essentially no other options are available to fill the void between optimizing topical therapy and oral isotretinoin. Because of the emergence of P acnes strains that are less sensitive to oral antibiotics, some patients may experience a diminished therapeutic response to antibiotic therapy. As a result, responsible use of antibiotic therapy is suggested, incorporating measures to reduce the risk for antibiotic resistance.[11,12,22]

Before prescribing an oral antibiotic, a complete medical history must be obtained. Considerations related to individual patients, such as history of hepatitis or renal insufficiency, may lead to avoidance of specific antibiotics because of relative contraindications or potential side effects. Experts have suggested that trimethoprim/sulfamethoxazole be avoided in patients who have folate deficiency or megaloblastic hematopoiesis.[57]

Obtaining a complete medication history, including prescription and over-the-counter medications, is also important at the initial visit and all follow-up visits, This information allows continued assessment of potentially significant food–drug interactions, which may lead to a poor therapeutic response, or drug–drug interactions, which may result in toxicity. Past history of other oral antibiotics and topical agents used to treat acne vulgaris is also important to ascertain. For patients who have a history of oral or topical antibiotic use, especially if recent or without concomitant use of benzoyl peroxide, it may be beneficial to suppress any existing antibiotic-resistant P acnes strains by having the patient initiate benzoyl peroxide use for 2 to 3 weeks before initiating oral antibiotic therapy.[12,35,37]

When prescribing an oral antibiotic for acne vulgaris, a viable approach is to use an optimized topical therapy program from the outset when initiating oral antibiotic therapy. This regimen would include a benzoyl peroxide–containing formulation, because of its proven ability to suppress emergence and proliferation of less-sensitive P acnes organisms, and a topical retinoid.[22,30,33,34,36,45] A "leave on" formulation of benzoyl peroxide (ie, gel, cream), with or without topical clindamycin, is optimal for facial use. Alternatively, a quality benzoyl peroxide cleanser or wash may be used, especially for truncal skin, in patients less tolerant to "leave on" benzoyl peroxide or those who exhibit poor compliance with application of multiple "leave on" products. Some benzoyl peroxide wash/cleanser formulations have been shown to reduce P acnes and have therapeutic activity.[35,59]

Furthermore, data from studies using doxycycline, azithromycin, and clarithromycin show that a marked increase in resistant bacteria develops within the first 1 to 2 weeks, and the emergence of clindamycin-resistant P acnes becomes apparent after 8 weeks of topical clindamycin application.[60–62] Although more data are needed, it is prudent to combine an appropriate topical regimen with oral antibiotic therapy initially to suppress antibiotic resistance and maximize therapeutic response.

This article includes several additional suggestions to optimize outcomes and reduce antibiotic resistance, including limiting the duration of oral antibiotic therapy if clinically feasible and re-treating with the same previously effective oral antibiotic.

Consideration of potential adverse reactions may influence oral antibiotic selection. The availability of extended-release minocycline 1 mg/kg administered once daily has been shown to reduce the risk for acute vestibular reactions compared with immediate-release minocycline, and allows for lower cumulative drug exposure because of its pharmacokinetic profile.[17,18,51] Although some agents may rarely be associated with major adverse reactions, patient education and informed consent are important issues to address before initiation of therapy.

SUMMARY

Oral antibiotic therapy is indicated for treatment of moderate to severe acne vulgaris and is optimally used in combination with a rational topical regimen.

The recommended treatment duration, if clinically feasible, is 3 to 6 months, with long-term maintenance achieved whenever possible with topical therapy. Because of a progressive increase in the emergence of antibiotic-resistant *P acnes* strains, some patients have experienced a decrease in therapeutic response over time. This finding has led to the development of suggested methods to reduce the risk for antibiotic resistance and preserve clinical benefit. Oral antibiotics used to treat acne vulgaris differ in their pharmacologic properties and adverse reaction potential. Treatment benefit may be maximized through rational antibiotic selection and use, coupled with appropriate patient follow-up.

REFERENCES

1. Weinstock MA, Boyle M. Statistics of interest to the dermatologist. In: Thiers BH, Lang PG, editors. Year book of dermatology. Philadelphia: Elsevier Mosby; 2007. p. 49.
2. James WD. Clinical practice. Acne. N Engl J Med 2005;352(14):1463–72.
3. Krakowski A, Eichenfield LF. Pediatric acne: clinical presentations, evaluation, and management. J Drugs Dermatol 2007;6(6):589–93.
4. Tan JK. Psychosocial impact of acne vulgaris: evaluating the evidence. Skin Therapy Lett 2004;9(7):1–3.
5. Rapp DA, Brenes GA, Feldman SR, et al. Anger and acne: implications for quality of life, patient satisfaction and clinical care. Br J Dermatol 2004;151(1):183–9.
6. Bruggemann H. Insights in the pathogenic potential of *Propionibacterium acnes* from its complete genome. Semin Cutan Med Surg 2005;24(2):63–72.
7. Harper JC. An update on the pathogenesis and management of acne vulgaris. J Am Acad Dermatol 2004;51(1):S36–8.
8. Rosen T. The *Propionibacterium acnes* genome: from the laboratory to the clinic. J Drugs Dermatol 2007;6(6):582–6.
9. McInturff JE, Kim J. The role of toll like receptors in the pathophysiology of acne. Semin Cutan Med Surg 2005;24(2):73–8.
10. Holland DB, Jeremy AH. The role of inflammation in the pathogenesis of acne and acne scarring. Semin Cutan Med Surg 2005;24(2):79–83.
11. Leyden JJ, Del Rosso JQ, Webster GF. Clinical considerations in the treatment of acne vulgaris and other inflammatory skin disorders. Cutis 2007; 79(6S):9–25.
12. Gollnick H, Cunliffe W, Berson D, et al. Management of acne: report from a global alliance to improve outcomes in acne. J Am Acad Dermatol 2003;49(1): S1–37.
13. Del Rosso JQ. A status report on the use of subantimicrobial-dose doxycycline: a review of the biologic and antimicrobial effects of the tetracyclines. Cutis 2004;74:118–22.
14. Webster GW, Del Rosso JQ. Anti-inflammatory activity of tetracyclines. Dermatol Clin 2007;25(2):133–5.
15. Del Rosso JQ. Report from the scientific panel on antibiotic use in dermatology: introduction. Cutis 2007;79(6S):6–8.
16. Del Rosso JQ. Update from the scientific panel on antibiotic use in dermatology: introduction. Cutis 2008; (manuscript in preparation).
17. Leyden JJ. Extended-release minocycline—first systemic antibiotic approved for the treatment of acne: introduction. Cutis 2006;78(4S):4–5.
18. Del Rosso JQ. Recently approved systemic therapies for acne vulgaris and rosacea. Cutis 2007; 80(2):113–20.
19. Bikowski JB. Subantimicrobial dose doxycycline for acne and rosacea. SkinMed 2003 July–August: 234–45.
20. Feldman S, Carrecia R, Barham KL, et al. Diagnosis and treatment of acne. Am Fam Physician 2004; 69(9):2123–30.
21. Haider A, Shaw JC. Treatment of acne vulgaris. JAMA 2004;292(6):726–35.
22. Tan AW, Tan HH. Acne vulgaris: a review of antibiotic therapy. Expert Opin Pharmacother 2005;6(3): 409–18.
23. Ross JI, Snelling AM, Eady EA, et al. Phenotypic and genotypic characterization of antibiotic-resistant Propionibacterium acnes isolated from acne patients attending dermatologic clinics in Europe, the USA, Japan and Australia. Br J Dermatol 2001;144:339–46.
24. Ross JI, Snelling AM, Carnegie E, et al. Antibiotic-resistant acne: lessons from Europe. Br J Dermatol 2003;148(3):467–78.

25. Eady AE, Cove JH, Layton AM. Is antibiotic resistance in cutaneous propionibacteria clinically relevant? Implications of resistance for acne patients and prescribers. Am J Clin Dermatol 2003;4: 813–31.

26. Amin K, Riddle CC, Aires DJ, et al. Common and alternative oral therapies for acne vulgaris : a review. J Drugs Dermatol 2007;6(9):873–80.

27. Bhambri S, Del Rosso JQ, Desai A. Oral trimethoprim-sulfamethoxazole in the treatment of acne vulgaris. Cutis 2007;79(6):430–4.

28. Rafiei R, Yaghoobi R. Azithromycin versus tetracycline in the treatment of acne vulgaris. J Drugs Dermatol 2006;17(14):217–21.

29. Leyden JJ. The evolving role of Propionibacterium acnes in acne. Semin Cutan Med Surg 2001;20: 139–43.

30. Leyden JJ. A review of the use of combination therapies for the treatment of acne vulgaris. J Am Acad Dermatol 2003;49(3):S206–10.

31. Tanghetti E. The impact and importance of resistance. Cutis 2007;80(1S):5–9.

32. Del Rosso JQ. Study results of benzoyl peroxide 5%/clindamycin 1% topical gel, adapalene 0.1% gel, and use in combination for acne vulgaris. J Drugs Dermatol 2007;6(6):616–22.

33. Lookingbill DP, Dhalker DK, Lindholm JS. Treatment of acne with a combination clindamycin/benzoyl peroxide gel compared with clindamycin gel, benzoyl peroxide gel and vehicle gel: combined results of two double-blind investigations. J Am Acad Dermatol 1997;37:590–5.

34. Leyden J, Kaidbey K, Levy S, et al. The combination formulation of clindamycin 1% plus benzoyl peroxide 5% versus 3 different formulations of topical clindamycin alone in the reduction of Propionibacterium acnes. Am J Clin Dermatol 2001;2:263–6.

35. Leyden JJ, Plott T, Wortzman M. Antibiotic-resistant P. acnes are suppressed by a 6% benzoyl peroxide wash. 31st Hawaii Dermatology Seminar. Wailea, Maui, Hawaii. March 3-9, 2007 [Poster].

36. Leyden JJ. Antibiotic resistance in the topical treatment of acne vulgaris. Cutis 2004;73(6S):6–9.

37. Eady EA, Farmery MR, Ross JL, et al. Effects of benzoyl peroxide and erythromycin alone and in combination against antibiotic-sensitive and -resistant skin bacteria from acne patients. Br J Dermatol 1994; 131(3):331–6.

38. Del Rosso JQ, Leyden JJ. Status report on antibiotic resistance: implications for the dermatologist. Dermatol Clin 2007;25(2):127–32.

39. Leyden JJ, McGinley KJ, Cavalieri S, et al. Propionibacterium acnes resistance to antibiotics in acne patients. J Am Acad Dermatol 1983;8(1):41–5.

40. Eady EA, Jones CE, Tipper JL, et al. Antibiotic resistant propionibacteria in acne: need for policies to modify antibiotic use. Br Med J 1993;306(6877):555–6.

41. Eady EA, Gloor M, Leyden JJ. Propionibacterium acnes resistance: a worldwide problem. Dermatology 2003;206(1):54–6.

42. Simpson N. Antibiotics in acne: time for a rethink. Br J Dermatol 2001;144(2):225–8.

43. Cooper AJ. Systematic review of Propionibacterium acnes resistance to systemic antibiotics. Med J Aust 1998;169(5):259–61.

44. Thevarajah S, Balkrishnan R, Camacho F, et al. Trends in prescription of acne medication in the US: shift from antibiotic to non-antibiotic treatment. J Dermatolog Treat 2005;16:224–8.

45. Tanghetti E. Antibiotic resistance and the role of combination acne therapy: introduction. Cutis 2007;80(1S):3.

46. Eady EA, Cove JH, Holland KT. Erythromycin resistant propionibacteria in antibiotic treated acne patients: association with therapeutic failure. Br J Dermatol 1989;121:51–7.

47. Ozolins M, Eady EA, Avery AJ, et al. Comparison of five antimicrobial regimens for treatment of mild to moderate facial acne vulgaris in the community: randomized controlled trial. Lancet 2004;364(9452): 2188–95.

48. Simonart T, Dramaix M. Treatment of acne with topical antibiotics: lessons from clinical studies. Br J Dermatol 2005;153:395–403.

49. Schlessinger J, Menter A, Gold M, et al. Clinical safety and efficacy studies of a novel formulation combining 1.2% clindamycin phosphate and 0.025% tretinoin for the treatment of acne vulgaris. J Drugs Dermatol 2007;6(6):607–15.

50. Shalita AR, Myers JA, Krochmal L, et al. The safety and efficacy of clindamycin phosphate foam 1% versus clindamycin topical gel 1% for the treatment of acne vulgaris. J Drugs Dermatol 2005;4:48–56.

51. Fleischer AB, Dinehart S, Stowe D, et al. Safety and efficacy of a new extended-release formulation of minocycline. Cutis 2006;78(4S):21–31.

52. Skidmore R, Kovach R, Walker C, et al. Effects of subantimicrobial-dose doxycycline in the treatment of moderate acne. Arch Dermatol 2003;139:459–64.

53. Cunliffe WJ, Aldana OL, Goulden V. Oral trimethoprim: a relatively safe and successful third-line treatment for acne vulgaris. Br J Dermatol 1999;141(4): 757–8.

54. Campbell JL. A comparative review of the efficacy and tolerability of retinoid-containing combination regimens for the treatment of acne vulgaris. J Drugs Dermatol 2007;6(6):625–9.

55. Del Rosso JQ. Systemic therapy for rosacea: focus on oral antibiotic therapy and safety. Cutis 2000; 66(4S):7–13.

56. Knowles SR, Shear SR. Cutaneous drug reactions associated with systemic features. In: Wolverton SE, editor. Comprehensive dermatologic

drug therapy. 2nd edition. Philadelphia: Saunders Elsevier; 2007. p. 977–83.

57. Remlinger KA. Hematologic toxicity of drug therapy. In: Wolverton SE, editor. Comprehensive dermatologic drug therapy. 2nd edition. Philadelphia: Saunders Elsevier; 2007. p. 901–3.

58. Feldman SR. The parable of the piano teacher. Skin and Aging. August 2007;6.

59. Del Rosso JQ. Keeping it clean: a look at the clinical benefits of newer formulations of therapeutic cleansers for acne, rosacea and seborrheic dermatitis. Skin and Aging. August 2003;83–8.

60. Walker C, Bradshaw M. The effect of oral doxycycline 100 mg once daily for 14 days on the nasopharyngeal flora of healthy volunteers: a preliminary analysis. Fall Clinical Dermatology, Las Vegas, Nevada, October 18–21, 2007 [Poster].

61. Malhotra-Kumar S, Lammens C, Coenen S, et al. Effect of azithromycin and clarithromycin therapy on pharyngeal carriage of macrolide resistant streptococci in healthy volunteers: a randomized, double-blind, placebo-controlled study. Lancet 2007;369: 482–90.

62. Cunliffe WJ, Holland KJ, Bojar R, et al. A randomized, double-blind comparison of a clindamycin phosphate/benzoyl peroxide gel formulation and a matching clindamycin gel with respect to microbiologic activity and clinical efficacy in the topical treatment of acne vulgaris. Clin Ther 2002;24(7): 1117–33.

How to Handle a CA-MRSA Outbreak

Dirk M. Elston, MD

KEYWORDS

• MRSA • Colonization abscess therapy

The incidence of infection with community-type strains of methicillin-resistant *Staphylococcus aureus* (CA-MRSA) continues to increase. Large CA-MRSA abscesses are now common in the dermatologist's office, and evidence suggests that MRSA strains are more virulent than methicillin-sensitive (MSSA) strains, as judged by worse outcomes and higher cost of care.[1] This article presents a practical approach to patients who have CA-MRSA infection and provides guidance on how to deal with community outbreaks.

EMERGING DATA ON INFECTIONS CAUSED BY COMMUNITY-TYPE STRAINS OF METHICILLIN-RESISTANT *STAPHYLOCOCCUS AUREUS*

Most cutaneous CA-MRSA infections present as folliculitis or spontaneous abscess with or without accompanying cellulitis. Uncomplicated CA-MRSA abscesses respond to drainage, and antibiotics are not needed in most cases. CA-MRSA abscesses commonly occur on the thighs, buttocks, flanks, head, and neck. Pediatric orbital cellulitis, once caused predominantly by *Haemophilus influenzae*, is now commonly caused by MRSA. Patients typically have an accompanying sinusitis.[2]

Although patients who have sepsis or necrotizing pneumonitis typically present with life-threatening manifestations, these rarely progress from simple skin infections to more serious systemic disease if managed properly. Furuncles represent small follicular abscesses, and abscesses large and small respond to drainage. This seems no less true for CA-MRSA abscesses than for those caused by other organisms. Antibiotics are often unnecessary after adequate surgical drainage of uncomplicated skin and soft tissue abscesses caused by CA- MRSA.[3–6] Reasons to avoid antibiotics when they are not needed include the risk for complications (eg, Stevens-Johnson syndrome, diarrhea) and the emergence of antibiotic resistance.

The key to effective management is early intervention with adequate drainage. A cruciate or punch incision is less likely to seal over and is preferred. A curette is useful to ensure that all loculated purulent material has been liberated and evacuated. Packing is generally best avoided, because purulent material can re-form rapidly behind the packing material. Drains and irrigation may be helpful to prevent reaccumulation of purulent material.

With proper surgical management, prognosis is excellent for most patients who have cutaneous MRSA infections. For those who require antibiotic therapy, most can be managed cost-effectively with sulfa or tetracyclines. Clindamycin remains useful in many areas of the country, although inducible resistance is emerging as an important problem. Reports of good outcomes with clindamycin in areas with high rates of inducible resistance are probably a reflection of adequate surgical drainage of the lesions.

Although CA-MRSA abscesses are often large and painful, overall prognosis is good when they are adequately drained. However, this projection is not cause for complacency, because furunculosis and abscess can occasionally lead to fatal complications, such as sepsis and pneumonitis. CA-MRSA pneumonitides, empyema, and osteomyelitis tend to affect children, and may be complicated by deep venous thrombosis, pulmonary embolus, hemophagocytic syndrome, or rapidly progressive glomerulonephritis.[7,8]

The risk for a severe complication in the index patient or a close contact has prompted some

No relevant conflict of interest. The author has been a consultant for Abbott, Medicis, and Collagenix.
Department of Dermatology, Geisinger Medical Center, 100 North Academy Avenue, Danville, PA 17822, USA
E-mail address: dmelston@geisinger.edu

Dermatol Clin 27 (2009) 43–48
doi:10.1016/j.det.2008.07.005

authorities to suggest decolonization of all infected patients and their immediate contacts. This subject is highly controversial, and it should be noted that decolonization of clinically infected patients is different from routine screening of the population with decolonization of those who have positive cultures but no clinical signs or symptoms. Emerging evidence continues to support decolonization of infected patients and their contacts in some clinical situations. Some evidence supports screening of patients on hospital admission. However, little evidence supports routine screening of the entire population or attempts to eradicate the organism nationally.

Just how common is colonization of close contacts? In a Swedish study, MRSA was found to spread to family members in 43% (22/51) of the families studied. Among the families with spread, 70% (42/60) of household contacts were positive for MRSA. Transmission occurred among adult couples, parents and children, grandparents and children, and siblings, suggesting that limited physical contact can spread the organism.[9]

EMERGING RESISTANCE PATTERNS

The routine use of antibiotics in livestock seems to be contributing to the emergence of resistant organisms. In a study in the Netherlands, 11% of pigs from 31 farms were colonized with MRSA in their nares, and routine antibiotic use was a risk factor for MRSA carriage. Pigs from all but one of the 6 farms supplying pigs for the MRSA-positive farms were MRSA positive. Isolated strains were found to contain either staphylococcal chromosomal cassette mec (SCCmec) type IV or V, but type V was predominant. All of the isolated strains were resistant to tetracycline, and additional resistances included erythromycin, lincomycin, kanamycin, and gentamicin.[10]

EFFECT OF RESISTANCE PATTERNS ON CHOICE OF THERAPY

Surgical drainage remains the most important intervention for most CA-MRSA infections. Thus, in many instances, emerging resistance patterns will have little effect on outcome. Their main effect may be to emphasize that antibiotics should be used responsibly and only when necessary to stem the emergence of resistant strains.

A randomized, double-blind trial of 166 outpatient subjects compared placebo with cephalexin, 500 mg, orally four times for 7 days in patients who had skin and soft tissue abscesses. All patients underwent incision and drainage of their lesions. *Staphylococcus aureus* was isolated from 70.4%

of the abscess cultures, and 87.8% of the isolates tested showed MRSA. Panton-Valentine leukocidin (PVL) genes were present in 93% of the isolates. The groups showed no significant difference in the clinical cure rate (90.5% vs. 84.1%, $P = .25$), suggesting that antibiotics may be unnecessary after adequate surgical drainage of uncomplicated skin and soft tissue abscesses caused by CA-MRSA.[3] A retrospective review of 245 children who underwent incision and drainage of neck abscesses in 2005 showed that the incidence of MRSA increased from 9% to 40% during the 1-year study period, but the clinical course of infection did not appear different.[11]

Clindamycin resistance is emerging as a significant problem but is highly regional. Despite a significant increase in empiric clindamycin use, one study of 296 S aureus skin and soft tissue infections showed that 97% of the CA-MRSA isolates retained susceptibility to clindamycin. In the study, 73% of isolates were MRSA, of which 87% were CA-MRSA.[12] In other areas, resistance rates are much higher,[13,14] which is a particular problem, because clindamycin has been one of the better oral agents for clearance of nasal carriage.

Inducible clindamycin resistance seems to be more common among patients who have cystic fibrosis. Of 703 patients who had MRSA, 48% (68/143) of those who had cystic fibrosis had at least one isolate with inducible resistance compared with 8% (43/560) of the patients who did not have cystic fibrosis ($P < .01$). Inducible resistance was also more common among MSSA isolated from patients who had cystic fibrosis. Inducible resistance was found in at least one isolate from 29% (73/254) of the patients who had cystic fibrosis versus 17% (88/508) of those who did not have cystic fibrosis ($P < .01$).[15] Therefore, clindamycin may be a poor empiric antibiotic choice in children who have cystic fibrosis and a skin or soft tissue infection.

Therapeutic failure with vancomycin has been associated with intracellular survival of bacteria within leukocytes. An in vitro study comparing various antimicrobial regimens (vancomycin, linezolid, quinupristin/dalfopristin, arbekacin with and without rifampicin plus sulfamethoxazole/trimethoprim) showed that although vancomycin killed 99% of extracellular MRSA, it was associated with one of the highest intracellular survival ratios (33.8%). Adding rifampicin with or without sulfamethoxazole/trimethoprim resulted in survival ratios of 0.78% and 1.02%, respectively. Combination therapy did not add to the intracellular killing for linezolid, quinupristin/dalfopristin, or arbekacin.[16]

Linezolid can be effective in the treatment of multidrug-resistant MRSA even when concentrations at the infection site are compromised by impaired blood flow. In six patients who had severe peripheral vascular disease and diabetic foot infections, concentrations in tissue were 18% to 78% of serum concentrations but were able to achieve bactericidal activity for at least half of the dosing interval against four of the five strains isolated.[17]

Telavancin is a novel multivalent lipoglycopeptide with rapid bactericidal activity against CA-MRSA.[18] In vitro evidence suggests that it will be a valuable addition to the armamentarium.

EVIDENCE SUPPORTING DECOLONIZATION OF INFECTED PATIENTS IN SOME CLINICAL SETTINGS

Many of these studies were conducted in hospital and chronic care settings, rather than in the community. CA-MRSA strains are increasingly prevalent in these settings, but hospital-type strains are also prevalent. The studies presented represent the best data currently available. This area is rapidly evolving and some conclusions may change as more data emerge.

Chlorhexidine bathing and intranasal mupirocin therapy was effective in decreasing the incidence of MRSA colonization and clinical infection among patients in the intensive care unit (ICU) who were colonized with MRSA. Treatment resulted in a 52% decrease in the infection rate ($P = .048$). However, in this particular hospital, all MRSA isolates were susceptible to chlorhexidine and the rate of mupirocin resistance was only 4.4%. Resistance did not increase during the period studied.[19]

A Brazilian study evaluated the efficacy of a program to prevent the spread of MRSA in an ICU. Measures included educational programs, early identification of patients infected or colonized with MRSA, contact isolation, and treatment of nasal carriage with topical mupirocin. Infection rates in the control, intervention, and postintervention groups were 10.2, 5.1, and 2.5 per 1000 patients per day ($P < .001$) with a reduction in mortality.[20]

Environmental contamination with MRSA was found to be common in a study of 2436 environmental samples from an ICU. Although the finding is concerning, this particular study found that transmission of MRSA from the environment to patients was not common.[21] Future studies should address this point to determine the appropriate targets for decolonization: the patient, care providers, other patients in the unit, visitors, or their contacts. The data presented earlier suggest that a fairly narrow target including the patient and their contacts and caregivers who have signs and symptoms may be appropriate.

A cluster randomized, double-blind, placebo-controlled trial of targeted intranasal mupirocin therapy in soldiers colonized with CA-MRSA failed to prevent infection in treated individuals and to prevent new colonization and infection within the study groups. The rate of mupirocin resistance was not assessed, nor was any strategy used to address MRSA colonization of any site other than the nose. This study showed that 5 of 65 soldiers (7.7%) treated with placebo and 7 of 66 (10.6%) treated with mupirocin developed clinical infections. Among those not initially colonized with CA-MRSA, 63 of 1459 (4.3) of the placebo group and 56 of 1607 (3.5%) of the mupirocin-treated group developed clinical infections.[22] This study suggests that population-based interventions that address only nasal carriage may do little to stem the spread of disease.

The Dutch ascribe their low prevalence of infection and colonization with MRSA to a national "search-and-destroy" policy, but this policy focuses on patients who have clinical signs and symptoms rather than mass screening of the population. Official guidelines from the Netherlands are simple and do not grade level of evidence; this is also true of New Zealand's guidelines. Guidelines from Germany, North America, Ireland, and the United Kingdom grade strength of evidence, but epidemiologic data suggest that guidelines based on higher level of evidence do not translate to lower rates of infection.[23]

Additional methods to control the spread of colonization within hospitals include developing an electronic signal to identify patients who are MRSA-positive, strict isolation of patients who are MRSA-positive, screening of patients at readmission or discharge, and screening of contacts.[24] Some programs have integrated all of these interventions. Although this strategy is likely not necessary in all settings, well-designed integrated screening and eradication programs may be appropriate for high-risk hospital settings.

Recurrence and spread of CA-MRSA infections may be related to persistent colonization, a colonized contact, or contaminated fomites. The colonized contact may be a human, pet, or farm animal. For decolonization to be successful, both nasal and skin surface colonization must be addressed. Among athletes, sharing of a towel or soap has been has been identified as a risk factor for MRSA infection during an outbreak. In suburban homes, children commonly share a bathroom that may have only one or two towel bars, which represent an important route of infection for siblings. A simple intervention is to replace bar soap with liquid soap. Each child should have a towel, which should be removed from the bathroom and hung over a chair to dry rather than remain in the bathroom where it may be used by a sibling.

Oral and intravenous antibiotics used for MRSA infection achieve poor levels on the skin surface, so systemic therapy alone allows colonization to persist. Topical agents such as chlorhexidine, triclosan, or Dakin's solution (dilute bleach) have been useful in addressing skin surface colonization. Rubbing alcohol or alcohol-based hand sterilizers can be used to wipe down fomites, such as wrestling mats and shoulder pads that can be damaged by bleach.

Resistance to topical antimicrobials is emerging as a serious problem. Over-the-counter (OTC) availability of triclosan in consumer products is likely to contribute to the emergence of resistance, and restrictions on OTC sales should be considered. Emerging evidence of resistance to topical antimicrobials will be covered in more detail in a separate article.

Parents often ask advice about preventing CA-MRSA infections during an outbreak. Athletes are at particular risk, partly because they are subject to minor skin injuries that serve as portals of entry. Routine use of chlorhexidine or triclosan to prevent infection will certainly contribute to the emergence of resistance, as can chronic antimicrobial use for chronic wounds or chronically colonized eczemas. If chlorhexidine and triclosan are abused in this setting, they will be lost as valuable agents.

Alternatives to prevent colonization in high-risk individuals include dilute bleach baths, benzoyl peroxide, and zinc compounds. Agents such as dilute bleach (2 tablespoons per tub of water) show little potential for emergence of resistance. Benzoyl peroxide soaps or washes may also be valuable in preventing colonization and are easier to use; studies are needed to validate their role. Zinc compounds such as zinc pyrithione are also promising; rather than exerting a bacteriocidal effect, they seem to interfere with bacterial adherence.

Mupirocin resistance is becoming increasingly common and has been linked to failure to eradicate MRSA colonization. A cluster of skin and soft tissue infections caused by a CA-MRSA strain identical to USA400 has occurred in Canada. An important finding was that more than 50% of the isolates had high-level resistance to mupirocin.[25] In other areas, resistance rates are much lower, but the emergence of mupirocin resistance is a disturbing trend.

The success rate for a single attempt at decolonization is disappointing. A double-blind, placebo-controlled 5-day trial of mupirocin for the anterior nares together with chlorhexidine soap for the skin was successful in only 25% of patients in the mupirocin group compared with an even poorer 18% in the group using chlorhexidine alone. However, fomites such as bar soap and towels were not addressed in this study. Low-level mupirocin resistance was associated with treatment failure ($P = .003$).[26] Another study compared a "pharmacologic regimen" of mupirocin 2% nasal ointment, chlorhexidine gluconate 4% soap, and silver sulfadiazine 1% cream with a "natural regimen" consisting of 5% tea tree oil body wash and 10% cream tea tree oil cream. Clearance rates were similar (49% vs. 41%).

When addressing a MRSA outbreak, it is helpful to have an easy to remember checklist of steps to eliminate colonization and address issues of reexposure to the pathogen. **Box 1** provides a helpful mnemonic for items that must be addressed.

Box 1
How to handle a methicillin-resistant
Staphylococcus aureus **outbreak in the office**

Address the **GAPS IN CARE**

  <u>G</u>roin

  <u>A</u>xillae

  <u>P</u>erianal

  <u>S</u>kin folds

  <u>I</u>solation

  <u>N</u>ares

  <u>C</u>uts

  <u>A</u>brasions

  <u>R</u>oom, daycare, and sport fomites

  <u>E</u>czematous skin

- Address colonization of the

  -<u>G</u>roin

  -<u>A</u>xillae

  -<u>P</u>erianal region

  -<u>S</u>kin folds

- Address the issue of

  -<u>I</u>solation

- Address colonization of the

  -<u>N</u>ares

- Address risk factors for colonization and infection

  -<u>C</u>uts

  -<u>A</u>brasions

  -<u>R</u>oom, daycare, and sport fomites

  -<u>E</u>czematous skin

Agents helpful in eliminating colonization of nares include clindamycin, rifampin/minocycline, mupirocin, retapamulin, gentamycin, and neomycin. Agents that can eliminate colonization on the skin include chlorhexidine, triclosan, ethanol, Dakin's solution, benzoyl peroxide, zinc, silver sufadiazine, and silver nitrate.

The most frequent site of colonization in the nares is the anterior nasal vestibule toward the very tip of the nose. This area has the highest yield for culture and must be addressed when topical agents are applied. Culture yield is higher if the swab is moistened slightly with the transport medium before collection. The swab should be carried forward to the anterior portion of the nare.

MRSA on fomites such as keyboards, toys, wrestling mats, and shoulder pads can be eliminated through washing, rubbing down with ethanol, or treating with a chlorhexidine or triclosan-based hand-sterilizer in an alcohol vehicle. Various skin washes and alcohol-based hand sterilizers are commercially available.

There are several major challenges to controlling MRSA infections:

- Emerging resistance to oral and topical agents
- Oral and intravenous antibiotics achieve poor levels on the skin surface
- Fomites may be difficult to sterilize
- Limited numbers of examination rooms in offices that treat patients infected MRSA and also perform surgery

Handwashing remains a simple but often neglected step in the prevention of infectious diseases. Although leave-on hand disinfectants are helpful in reducing MRSA transmission, they have limited efficacy against other important emerging pathogens, such as community strains of *Clostridium difficile*, and cannot replace handwashing. Ethanol-based disinfectants can be used to clean soiled office fomites but cannot replace sterilization of surgical equipment.

REFERENCES

1. Shorr AF. Epidemiology and economic impact of methicillin-resistant staphylococcus aureus: review and analysis of the literature. Pharmacoeconomics 2007;25(9):751–68.

2. McKinley SH, Yen MT, Miller AM, et al. Microbiology of pediatric orbital cellulitis. Am J Ophthalmol 2007; 144(4):497–501.

3. Rajendran PM, Young D, Maurer T, et al. Randomized, double-blind, placebo-controlled trial of cephalexin for treatment of uncomplicated skin abscesses in a population at risk for community methicillin-resistant Staphylococcus aureus infection. Antimicrob Agents Chemother 2007;51(11):4044–8.

4. Fridkin SK, Hageman JC, Morrison M, et al. Active bacterial core surveillance program of the emerging infections program network. methicillin-resistant Staphylococcus aureus disease in three communities. N Engl J Med 2005;352(14):1436–44.

5. Lee MC, Rios AM, Aten MF, et al. Management and outcome of children with skin and soft tissue abscesses caused by community-acquired methicillin-resistant Staphylococcus aureus. Pediatr Infect Dis J 2004;23(2):123–7.

6. Young DM, Harris HW, Charlebois ED, et al. An epidemic of methicillin-resistant Staphylococcus aureus soft tissue infections among medically underserved patients. Arch Surg 2004;139(9):947–51.

7. Hoshino C, Satoh N, Sugawara S, et al. Community-acquired Staphylococcus aureus pneumonia accompanied by rapidly progressive glomerulonephritis and hemophagocytic syndrome. Intern Med 2007;46(13):1047–53.

8. Nourse C, Starr M, Munckhof W. Community-acquired methicillin-resistant Staphylococcus aureus causes severe disseminated infection and deep venous thrombosis in children: literature review and recommendations for management. J Paediatr Child Health 2007;43(10):656–61.

9. Johansson PJ, Gustafsson EB, Ringberg H. High prevalence of MRSA in household contacts. Scand J Infect Dis 2007;39(9):764–8.

10. van Duijkeren E, Ikawaty R, Broekhuizen-Stins MJ, et al. Transmission of methicillin-resistant Staphylococcus aureus strains between different kinds of pig farms. Vet Microbiol 2007;128(1–2):213–5.

11. Thomason TS, Brenski A, McClay J, et al. The rising incidence of methicillin-resistant Staphylococcus aureus in pediatric neck abscesses. Otolaryngol Head Neck Surg 2007;137(3):459–64.

12. Szczesiul JM, Shermock KM, Murtaza UI, et al. No decrease in clindamycin susceptibility despite increased use of clindamycin for pediatric community-associated methicillin-resistant staphylococcus aureus skin infections. Pediatr Infect Dis J 2007; 26(9):852–4.

13. Seal JB, Moreira B, Bethel CD, et al. Antimicrobial resistance in Staphylococcus aureus at the University of Chicago Hospitals: a 15-year longitudinal assessment in a large university-based hospital. Infect Control Hosp Epidemiol 2003;24(6):403–8.

14. Tsuji BT, Rybak MJ, Cheung CM, et al. Community- and health care-associated methicillin-resistant Staphylococcus aureus: a comparison of molecular epidemiology and antimicrobial activities of various agents. Diagn Microbiol Infect Dis 2007;58(1):41–7.

15. Moore ZS, Jerris RC, Hilinski JA. High prevalence of inducible clindamycin resistance among

Staphylococcus aureus isolates from patients with cystic fibrosis. J Cyst Fibros 2007;7(3):206–9.

16. Yamaoka T. The bactericidal effects of anti-MRSA agents with rifampicin and sulfamethoxazole-trimethoprim against intracellular phagocytized MRSA. J Infect Chemother 2007;13(3):141–6.

17. Stein GE, Schooley S, Peloquin CA, et al. Linezolid tissue penetration and serum activity against strains of methicillin-resistant Staphylococcus aureus with reduced vancomycin susceptibility in diabetic patients with foot infections. J Antimicrob Chemother 2007;60(4):819–23.

18. Saravolatz LD, Pawlak J, Johnson LB. Comparative activity of telavancin against isolates of community-associated methicillin-resistant Staphylococcus aureus. J Antimicrob Chemother 2007; 60(2):406–9.

19. Ridenour G, Lampen R, Federspiel J, et al. Selective use of intranasal mupirocin and chlorhexidine bathing and the incidence of methicillin-resistant staphylococcus aureus colonization and infection among intensive care unit patients. Infect Control Hosp Epidemiol 2007;28(10):1155–61.

20. Moreira M, Freitas MR, Martins ST, et al. Efficacy of a program of prevention and control for methicillin-resistant Staphylococcus aureus infections in an intensive-care unit. Braz J Infect Dis 2007;11(1): 57–62.

21. Wilson AP, Hayman S, Whitehouse T, et al. Importance of the environment for patient acquisition of methicillin-resistant staphylococcus aureus in the intensive care unit: a baseline study. Crit Care Med 2007;35(10):2275–9.

22. Ellis MW, Griffith ME, Dooley DP, et al. Targeted Intranasal mupirocin to prevent community-associated methicillin-resistant Staphylococcus aureus colonization and infection in soldiers: a cluster randomized controlled trial. Antimicrobial Agents Chemother 2007;51(10):3591–8.

23. Humphreys H. National guidelines for the control and prevention of methicillin-resistant Staphylococcus aureus-what do they tell us? Clin Microbiol Infect 2007;13(9):846–53.

24. van Trijp MJ, Melles DC, Hendriks WD, et al. Successful control of widespread methicillin-resistant Staphylococcus aureus colonization and infection in a large teaching hospital in the Netherlands. Infect Control Hosp Epidemiol 2007;28(8): 970–5.

25. Mulvey MR, MacDougall L, Cholin B, et al. Saskatchewan CA-MRSA Study Group. Community-associated methicillin-resistant Staphylococcus aureus, Canada. Emerging Infect Dis 2005;11(6): 844–50.

26. Harbarth S, Dharan S, Liassine N, et al. Randomized, placebo-controlled, double-blind trial to evaluate the efficacy of mupirocin for eradicating carriage of methicillin-resistant Staphylococcus aureus. Antimicrobial Agents Chemother 1999;43(6): 1412–6.

Antibiotic Use in Sexually Transmissible Diseases

Ted Rosen, MD[a,b,*], Travis Vandergriff, MD[a,b], Mandy Harting, MD[a,b]

KEYWORDS

• STD • Syphilis • Gonorrhea • LGV • Donovanosis

Dermatologists have historically played a major role in the diagnosis and treatment of sexually transmissible diseases (STDs) because many present with either characteristic or pathognomonic cutaneous manifestations. Although "syphilology" is no longer one of the key elements of everyday clinical practice, dermatologists continue to provide assistance to gynecologists, urologists, infectious disease specialists, and family physicians because of their expert dermatologic training in devising differential diagnosis for anogenital lesions.

Despite steadily improving public awareness and continued diagnostic and therapeutic advances, STDs remain a significant cause of acute and chronic morbidity and mortality worldwide.[1,2] According to a World Health Organization estimate, more than 300 million people are infected annually by curable sexually transmitted infections (AIDS excluded).[3] The full impact on public health runs the spectrum from painful adenopathy and dysuria to infertility and cervical neoplasia. Genital ulcers associated with many common bacterial and viral STDs also facilitate the transmission or acquisition of HIV and that some ulcerative STDs (notably genital herpes) may adversely affect the course of HIV infection.[4–6] As summarized in a recent review, even nonulcerative STDs may facilitate HIV acquisition through recruiting target immune effector cells into HIV-susceptible genital epithelium.[7] Yet another compelling reason for timely diagnosis and therapy of common STDs is the potential for a concomitant reduction in the risk for HIV transmission and acquisition.[6,8,9]

In addition to the cost in human suffering, STDs contribute an incredible economic burden to a global society still trying to cope with critical issues such as nuclear proliferation, pollution and climate change, emerging infectious diseases, war, famine and displaced populations.[10] The Centers for Disease Control and Prevention (CDC) estimated the direct health care costs for STDs at more than $13 billion annually in the United States alone.[11] However, this estimate is a 3 years old, and therefore the annual cost of care for STDs in America is probably even greater now, considering the slow but steady increase in incidence and prevalence of most STDs.

Considering the many long- and short-term individual and societal consequences of STDs enumerated above, health care providers must remain apprised of current trends in epidemiology, diagnosis, and management of these diseases. Thus, it is not unreasonable to expect dermatologists to have at least a working knowledge of current STD therapy. In concordance with the theme of this issue of *Dermatologic Clinics*, this article focuses on current diagnostic and therapeutic recommendationsr the classic STDs that have prominent cutaneous findings and would be treated with drugs belonging to the antibiotic class. These STDs include syphilis, chancroid, lymphogranuloma venereum, granuloma inguinale, gonorrhea, and genital bite wounds. Although chlamydial infections (urethritis, cervicitis) and bacterial vaginosis are also treated with antibiotics, these disorders are not managed by dermatologists and therefore are not discussed. **Table 1**

a Department of Dermatology, Baylor College of Medicine, 1 Baylor Plaza, Houston, TX 77030, USA
b Dermatology Service, Michael E. DeBakey VA Medical Center, 2002 Holcombe, Houston, TX 77030, USA
* Corresponding author.
E-mail address: vampireted@aol.com (T. Rosen).

Dermatol Clin 27 (2009) 49–61
doi:10.1016/j.det.2008.07.002
0733-8635/08/$ – see front matter. Published by Elsevier Inc.

Table 1
Antibiotics and sexually transmissible diseases

Disease State	Preferred Drug	Second-Line Drugs	Not Recommended
Syphilis	Benzathine penicillin G	Doxycycline Tetracycline	Azithromycin (dose uncertain) Ceftriaxone dose uncertain)
Chancroid	Azithromycin Ceftriaxone	Ciprofloxacin Erythromycin	Penicillins
Lymphogranuloma venereum	Doxycycline Minocycline	Erythromycin	Azithromycin Fluoroquinolones Sulfa drugs
Granuloma inguinale	Trimethoprim-sulfamethoxazole	Azithromycin Ciprofloxacin Erythromycin Aminoglycosides (most toxic option)	Doxycycline (regional variability)[b] Ceftriaxone (dose uncertain)[b]
Gonorrhea[a] (uncomplicated)	Ceftriaxone Cefixime	Spectinomycin Azithromycin (gastrointestinal upset)[b]	Erythromycin Fluoroquinolones (losing efficacy) Penicillins Tetracyclines
Gonorrhea[a] (disseminated)	Ceftriaxone Cefotaxime Ceftizoxime	Spectinomycin	Erythromycin Fluoroquinolones (losing efficacy) Penicillins Tetracyclines
Genital bite wound	Amoxicillin-clavulanic acid	Cefuroxime	Limited data

[a] Concomitant treatment for *Chlamydia trachomatis* should be considered.
[b] Uncertainty exists.

provides a broad overview of antibiotic use per disease.

SYPHILIS
Epidemiology

The protean and varied manifestations of syphilis earned this disease the well-deserved designation of "the great imitator," and led Sir William Osler to state that "Syphilis simulates every other disease. It is the only disease necessary to know."[12] Since its probable origin in the Western Hemisphere some 8000 years ago, syphilis continues to be a significant disorder, with worldwide incidence exceeding 12 million cases yearly.[13] The disease is most prevalent in developing countries, where up to 10% of the population may be infected. The rate of primary and secondary syphilis in the United States declined nearly 90% from 1990 to 2000, ultimately reaching an all-time low; however, this trend has steadily reversed, and latest statistics show that the reported incidence rate of primary and secondary syphilis has increased 57% since 2001, currently standing at 3.3 per 100,000 population.[14]

The recent resurgence of syphilis can be largely attributed to cases in men, with most occurring in men who have sex with men (MSM). Since 2000, for example, the incidence of syphilis in American men increased more than 70%, with similar developments in Europe and Canada.[15] One plausible theory suggests that this trend is caused by increased risky sexual behavior as individuals have become less fearful of HIV with the advent of highly active antiretroviral therapy (HAART). Equally important increases in syphilis rates have also occurred among inner-city, heterosexual African Americans of both genders.[14] Although the United States has had plans to eliminate syphilis since 1999, accomplishing this has obviously been more difficult than originally envisioned.[16]

Clinical Presentation and Diagnosis

Syphilis is caused by the spirochete *Treponema pallidum*, and the infection is directly transmitted through sexual contact (and transplacentally). Although the clinical manifestations of syphilis in adults have traditionally been divided into three distinct stages, these may have considerable overlap and serve mostly to simplify classification of presenting signs and symptoms.

The first stage, *primary syphilis*, is characterized by the chancre, a lesion that develops at the site of inoculation 9 to 90 days after exposure (most often 14–21 days). The chancre begins as an erythematous, painless papule 0.5 to 2 cm in diameter that eventually ulcerates. The chancre is characterized by a clean base with indurated, rolled borders and a characteristic "punched-out" appearance. The remarkably painless ulcer may be accompanied by moderate, painless, bilateral inguinal adenopathy.

When the chancre appears on the penis or scrotum in men or on the vulva or at the vaginal introitus in women, the ulcer is usually obvious, facilitating diagnosis at an early state. However, when occurring within the vaginal canal, anorectal region, or oropharynx, it may go unnoticed by the patient. Occult chancres are common in women and MSM, and the disease is typically not diagnosed until later in the disease course.[17] Regardless of location, chancres typically persist for 3 to 6 weeks and resolve spontaneously. In untreated patients, the treponemes proliferate and migrate through the lymphatic channels to the bloodstream where they disseminate. Metastatic accumulations of treponemes create the lesions characteristic of the second stage of syphilis.

Secondary syphilis is characterized by several signs and symptoms. Because the lesions appear 4 to 10 weeks after the primary chancre, some potential exists for overlap between the two stages. Currently, a persistent chancre along with clinically obvious secondary syphilis is highly suggestive of HIV coinfection.[18] More than 90% of patients who have secondary syphilis have skin or mucous membrane involvement. Although patients first develop a transient macular erythema involving the trunk and extremities, they later show the more characteristic copper-hued papulosquamous eruption involving the palms, soles, and trunk and may also have shallow erosions on oral mucous membranes (*mucous patches*).

When the scalp is involved, a noncicatricial, patchy, or "moth-eaten" alopecia ensues. Another potential sign of secondary syphilis is condyloma lata, which are smooth and moist, white to gray-colored, flat-topped, and globoid-shaped papules or plaques occurring in aggregates located in intertriginous areas. Additionally, patients may have systemic symptoms associated with secondary syphilis, such as low-grade fever, diffuse lymphadenopathy, malaise, fatigue, myalgia and arthralgia, anorexia, and weight loss. The signs and symptoms of secondary syphilis also resolve spontaneously without treatment. Untreated patients enter a latent stage during which treponemes continue to proliferate while the patient remains asymptomatic.

From the latent state, one third of untreated patients will ultimately develop late sequelae or tertiary syphilis. This stage begins approximately 3 to 15 years after initial infection, and associated complications are responsible for most syphilitic mortalities. Cardiovascular complications include stenosis of the coronary artery ostia and aortic root aneurysm leading to aortic insufficiency. Central nervous system tertiary syphilis may lead to altered mental status, focal neurologic deficits, tabes dorsalis, blindness, seizures, dementia, or psychosis. Persons coinfected with HIV are at increased risk for developing tertiary neurosyphilis.[19] The characteristic skin lesion of tertiary syphilis is the *gumma*, a necrotic granulomatous ulcer with indurated dusky-red serpiginous borders. Similar locally destructive lesions may also occur in the cartilage, bone, and brain.

In its primary stage, syphilis must be distinguished from other causes of genital ulcers, including STDs, invasive squamous cell carcinoma, and Behçet's disease. A definitive diagnosis of syphilis can be made in the primary stage by identifying treponemes using darkfield microscopy, a technique with few false-negative results and virtually no false-positive results. Alternatively, the exudate may be tested with direct fluorescent antibody (DFA) assays when available.

Serologic tests may also be used in primary syphilis, but results must be interpreted cautiously. The nontreponemal tests include the rapid plasma reagin (RPR) and venereal disease research laboratory (VDRL) tests, which measure antibody to cardiolipin ratios and are equally valid. The treponemal tests, including the fluorescent treponemal antibody absorption test (FTA-ABS) and microhemagglutination assay for *T pallidum* antibodies (MHA-TP), measure antibodies to specific treponemal proteins.

Within 1 week of chancre development, the nontreponemal tests are positive in approximately 85% of patients who have primary syphilis, but usually in titers lower than 1:16. Additionally, false-positive results are possible, and are most often associated with autoimmune disease, collagen vascular disease, HIV infection, tuberculosis, pregnancy, rickettsial infection, or bacterial endocarditis. The treponemal tests are positive in 90% of patients who have primary syphilis. Because most patients who have reactive FTA-ABS and MHA-TP assays remain reactive unless the disease is treated early in the primary stage, these specific treponemal tests are of limited use in diagnosing infection, but a negative result may exclude the diagnosis or confirm a suspected false-positive result on nontreponemal tests.

The cutaneous findings of secondary syphilis must be distinguished from primary HIV infection, other viral exanthems, lichen planus and psoriasis, pityriasis rosea, erythema multiforme, and drug eruptions. In the secondary stage, serologic tests become more reliable, with treponemal and nontreponemal assays routinely yielding positive results. Nontreponemal assays are positive in higher titers, often exceeding 1:64. A fourfold increase in titer presumptively diagnoses active infection. Additionally, darkfield microscopy may identify spirochetes in the exudates from moist lesions of secondary syphilis. Although it is not necessary for diagnosis, histopathologic evaluation of biopsied tissue shows a polymorphous cellular infiltrate typically rich in plasma cells, macrophages, and lymphocytes. A positive VDRL testing of cerebrospinal fluid is highly specific for tertiary neurosyphilis.

Treatment

As with other STDs, practitioners should review the most current CDC recommendations[20] when treating patients who have syphilis. Parenterally administered penicillin G remains the preferred drug for treating syphilis in all stages. Recommended treatment for adults who have primary or secondary syphilis is a single intramuscular dose of 2.4 million units of benzathine penicillin G, and has been used for more than 5 decades to achieve clinical cure. Children and prepubertal adolescents who have acquired primary or secondary syphilis should be evaluated for sexual abuse and treated with benzathine penicillin G in a single intramuscular dose of 50,000 units/kg, up to the adult dose of 2.4 million units. Pregnant women who have syphilis should be treated with the standard adult dose of benzathine penicillin G. Because of the risk for congenital syphilis, pregnant women allergic to penicillin should be desensitized and subsequently treated with penicillin in a controlled medical environment. Men and nonpregnant women who have penicillin allergy may be treated for primary, secondary, and early latent disease with doxycycline (100 mg orally twice daily for 14 days) or tetracycline (500 mg orally four times daily for 14 days).

The pain associated with benzathine penicillin injection, possibility of severe penicillin allergy, and protracted course of currently accepted alternative oral therapies have led experts to search for other single-dose or limited-duration treatments for early and incubating syphilis. Azithromycin, a macrolide with a long tissue half-life and efficacy in a rabbit model of syphilis, is one such agent. Although azithromycin administered in a single oral dose of 2 g has been equipotent to standard benzathine penicillin in some case series,[21–25] treatment failure has also been reported[26–28] and justifies caution when considering this drug. Failure of response to azithromycin is apparently caused by a single A→G mutation at position 2058 of the 23S rRNA gene of T pallidum; this mutation confers resistance through preventing macrolide binding to the bacterial 50S ribosomal subunit, of which 23S rRNA is a structural component.[28]

Another seemingly attractive therapy might be parenteral (intramuscular or intravenous) ceftriaxone. Although not single-dose, daily administration by a health care provider at least ensures patient compliance, and ceftriaxone is suitable for most patients who have penicillin allergy. In some immunocompetent patients, ceftriaxone has proven efficacious.[29,30] Unfortunately, the optimal dose and duration of this therapy is unknown, and clinicians have used doses ranging from 1.0 to 3.0 g in both single-dose and daily doses over variable periods ranging from 3 to 21 days.[31] Caution should certainly be used with patients coinfected with HIV, because serologic nonresponse and relapse may ensue.[32]

In the absence of active lesions (latent stage), patients are not contagious to sexual contacts, and treatment of latent syphilis does not reduce transmission to others but rather protects the patient against late sequelae. Treatment of latent syphilis may require a different dosing protocol. Patients who have latent syphilis who were infected within the past year are designated as *early latent syphilis* and should be treated with 2.4 million units of benzathine penicillin G in a single intramuscular dose. Patients who have latent syphilis lasting more than 1 year (or of unknown duration) should be treated with a total of 7.2 million units of benzathine penicillin G, administered in three intramuscular doses of 2.4 million units, with each dose separated by a 1 week interval. All patients who have tertiary syphilis should also be treated with the latter regimen.

Pregnant patients who have latent syphilis and known penicillin allergy should be desensitized and treated with penicillin. Nonpregnant patients who have early latent syphilis and penicillin allergy should be treated with the alternative regimens appropriate for primary and secondary syphilis. Patients who have late latent syphilis and penicillin allergy should receive either doxycycline (100 mg orally twice daily for 28 days) or tetracycline (500 mg orally four times daily for 28 days). Again, the benefit of azithormycin and ceftriaxone in later stages of syphilis is uncertain.

The management of syphilis in patients coinfected with HIV remains controversial. Although unusual serologic responses and atypical clinical lesions have been reported, most individuals have normal serologic and clinical features. Some concern exists that these individuals may be at increased risk for treatment failure, relapse, or neurosyphilis after standard therapeutic regimens. However, intensive treatment regimens do not seem to be more effective than routine therapy when used for the appropriate stage of infection.[33] Some authorities still recommend administering three weekly benzathine penicillin G injections to patients in early syphilis who are HIV coinfected, but this is not the current CDC recommendation.

Other Management Considerations

All patients should be warned about a possible Jarisch-Herxheimer reaction, which is an acute febrile reaction appearing within 12 hours of initial treatment for early stages of syphilis. Prophylactic antipyretic treatment has not been shown to prevent this phenomenon. Sex partners of patients diagnosed with syphilis should be clinically and serologically evaluated for syphilis and appropriately treated if necessary. Furthermore, individuals who have been exposed within 90 days before a sex partner is diagnosed with syphilis may have false-negative seroreactivity and should be treated for a presumptive diagnosis of syphilis.

Because of the high risk for concomitant infection, patients diagnosed with syphilis should always be evaluated for other STDs, including HIV. Treatment failure may occur with any regimen, and patients should be clinically and serologically reexamined 6 and 12 months after initial treatment. Patients who have persistent clinical signs or symptoms or a sustained fourfold increase in nontreponemal titers should be retreated and reevaluated for HIV infection.

CHANCROID
Epidemiology

In addition to syphilis, chancroid is a major cause of genital ulcer disease (GUD) worldwide. Although the diseases share some features, important differences exist in epidemiology, clinical presentation, diagnosis, and treatment, and the disorders were separated as distinct entities in the mid-19th century. In 1889, the specific causative bacillus was identified by an Italian dermatologist, Augusto Ducrey, after a series of experimental autoinoculations with ulcer material gathered from patients.[34] The etiologic microbe is thus deservedly dubbed *Haemophilus ducreyi*.

Because of irregularities in diagnostic accuracy and varying reporting practices, the exact global incidence of chancroid is unknown. Despite these uncertainties, many experts suspect that its worldwide incidence may actually surpass that of syphilis. In parts of sub-Saharan Africa, chancroid is the most common cause of GUD, and in India more than half of all genital ulcers are caused by chancroid.[34,35] Other endemic locales include the Caribbean basin and southern Asia. In the United States and other developed countries, chancroid occurs in discrete and sporadic outbreaks largely restricted to a few geographic areas.[36] Most recently reported American cases occurred in New York, North Carolina, South Carolina, and Texas, and the number of cases steadily declined from nearly 5000 in 1987 to just 143 in 1999. More recent CDC statistics suggest that chancroid is vanishing in the United States, with only 33 cases reported nationwide in 2006.[14] Prior American outbreaks affected mostly African American and Hispanic heterosexuals, with a male-to-female ratio ranging from 3:1 to 25:1. Commercial sex workers are important vectors of transmission worldwide, and outbreaks have also been associated with crack cocaine abuse.

Clinical Presentation and Diagnosis

Chancroid is caused by a gram-negative and facultative anaerobic coccobacillus. The bacterium enters skin through microabrasions created during intercourse. After a 4- to 7-day incubation period (longer in patients who have concomitant HIV infection), a tender erythematous papule or pustule develops at the inoculation site. Within days, a deep ulceration with central necrosis develops. The ulcer is characteristically spontaneously painful, tender to palpation, with soft, ragged, and undermined margins. A foul-smelling exudate and surrounding erythema are often present.

The ulcer appears in men most commonly on the prepuce and shaft of the penis, whereas in women they tend to occur on the labia and fourchette. Extragenital chancroid is rare. Approximately one half of patients develop painful unilateral or bilateral inguinal lymphadenopathy within several weeks.[37] Affected lymph nodes may become matted or fluctuant, eventually rupturing and forming suppurative tracts. Because of the propensity of chancroidal ulcers to autoinoculate adjacent skin, multiple opposing ulcerations ("kissing lesions") are characteristic. Untreated infections typically resolve spontaneously within 3 months, but potential complications include phimosis, local tissue destruction, and fistula formation. Less common clinical presentations of chancroid have also been described.[37,38]

In transient chancroid, the ulcer resolves in 4 to 6 days, and suppurative inguinal adenopathy develops weeks later. Follicular chancroid is characterized by ulcerations of the pilar apparatus in hair-bearing areas, such as at the base of the penis. Multiple small ulcerations coalesce to form a single ulcer that can cause considerable local destruction of tissue in the so-called "giant chancroid" variant.

Finally, phagedenic chancroid results in widespread necrosis and soft tissue destruction of genital or perigenital skin. A putative etiopathogenic factor has been recently characterized (*cytolethal distending factor*), which may account for the destructive and painful nature of the disease.[39]

Laboratory techniques for diagnosing chancroid are neither foolproof nor uniformly available. Gram stain of the ulcer debris may show the classic "school of fish" pattern of pleomorphic gram-negative coccobacilli in parallel chains or clusters. The definitive diagnosis requires isolation of *H ducreyi* on chocolate-based culture media (eg, gonococcal media) under conditions of high humidity and low oxygen tension.[40] However, even in experienced laboratories, the sensitivity of this technique is less than 80%. Nucleic acid amplification tests developed for research laboratories are the most sensitive and specific diagnostic assays but are not commercially available for routine diagnosis.[41] Because of somewhat suboptimal diagnostic modalities, the practical diagnosis of chancroid is based largely on clinical features. According to CDC recommendations, a likely diagnosis of chancroid can be made if all of the following criteria are met: (1) the patient has one or more painful genital ulcers; (2) darkfield examination of ulcer exudate or a serologic test for syphilis performed at least 7 days after onset of ulcers shows no evidence of *T pallidum* infection on; (3) the clinical presentation, appearance of genital ulcers, and, if present, regional lymphadenopathy are typical for chancroid; and (4) a test (viral culture or PCR) for herpes simplex virus performed on the ulcer exudate is negative.[14]

Treatment

Current CDC recommendations for chancroid therapy include the following regimens: azithromycin (1.0 g orally, administered as a single dose), ceftriaxone (single 250 mg intramuscular dose), ciprofloxacin (500 mg orally, twice daily, for three consecutive days), or erythromycin (500 mg orally, three times daily, for seven consecutive days). Azithromycin and ceftriaxone offer the benefit of single-dose therapy, eliminating the potential problem of noncompliance. Single-dose therapy may fail when patients are coinfected with HIV,[42,43] and synergistic combination antibiotic therapy (eg, streptomycin plus ceftriaxone) should be considered.[44] All routinely recommended regimens should be safe in pregnancy.

Although not yet commercialized for human use, a promising potential vaccine technology has been developed. In this scenario, high-risk individuals in endemic areas could undergo vaccination against a heme receptor essential for *H ducreyi* survival in skin. Antibodies arising after this vaccination have prevented infection in vivo in a porcine model of chancroid.[45]

Other Management Considerations

Patients diagnosed with chancroid should be tested for other STDs, including syphilis and HIV. In the United States, up to 10% of patients who have chancroid have concomitant syphilis. Patients should be reexamined 3 to 7 days after initiating therapy because failure to observe objective improvement in the ulcer suggests unsuccessful treatment. In these cases, one must consider whether the diagnosis of chancroid is correct, or if the patient has another confounding concomitant STD, including HIV, or if the *H ducreyi* isolate is drug-resistant. Suppurative lymph nodes heal more slowly than primary ulcers, and typically require needle aspiration to facilitate complete resolution.

LYMPHOGRANULOMA VENEREUM
Epidemiology

Differential diagnosis of GUD includes lymphogranuloma venereum (LGV), a disease that has recently received renewed attention because of its reemergence in developed countries. Caused by *Chlamydia trachomatis* serovars L1, L2, or L3, LGV has classically been a disease of tropical and subtropical climates. Endemic areas include India, Southeast Asia, South America, sub-Saharan Africa, and the Caribbean basin. Even in these areas, however, LGV is an uncommon cause of GUD, accounting for fewer than 10% of cases. In 2003, the first cases of LGV in Europe were documented in The Netherlands.[46–48] Since then, outbreaks have been reported throughout Europe, the United Kingdom, Australia, and both Canada and the United States.[49–53] Virtually all cases occurred in MSM and most often presented as acute proctitis or proctocolits, rather than as genital ulcers or inguinal adenopathy.

Common features in most of these reports, aside from MSM as the major demographic group affected, include Caucasian ethnicity, mean age older than 35 years, predominant (>70%) HIV coinfection, and concurrent sexually transmitted and hepatitis C infections.[54,55] Most also reported a large number of partners and repeated episodes of unprotected anal intercourse; the practice of "fisting" and use of sex toys were also reported.[54,55] Gene amplification techniques have identified the L2b strain of *C trachomatis* as the common variant in recent outbreaks in industrialized countries.[56] These techniques also determined that the L2b strain has been present in the United States since 1981, and that LGV has most likely been underdiagnosed during the past few decades. Recent cases might represent the discovery of a slow but ongoing epidemic rather than a novel outbreak.

Clinical Presentation and Diagnosis

LGV classically presents in three stages.[57] After an incubation period of 3 to 30 days, a small painless papule or herpetiform ulcer develops at the inoculation site. The primary ulcer resolves without treatment after 2 to 6 weeks, and most often goes unnoticed by the patient.[58]

The next stage of the disease is known as the *inguinal syndrome*, and is this stage at which most patients present for medical evaluation. LGV is predominantly a disease of the lymphatic tissue, and in the second stage, the nodes draining the site of inoculation enlarge and develop necrotic abscesses. Exquisitely painful regional lymph nodes may evolve into fluctuant buboes, which ultimately rupture in one third of patients. In men, adenopathy often involves the inguinal and femoral nodes. Prominent unilateral or bilateral inflammation of these nodes around the inguinal ligament create the so-called "groove sign," a finding considered to be pathognomonic for LGV. In women, however, only 20% to 30% develop inguinal adenopathy.[57] More commonly, the deep iliac and perirectal nodes are involved, because they drain the vaginal canal, cervix, rectum, and urethra.

Systemic symptoms, including fever, malaise, and arthralgia may be present in the second stage. Rare systemic complications have also been reported during the second stage and include pneumonitis, hepatitis, aseptic meningitis, and ocular inflammatory disease. The third stage is known as the genitoanorectal stage and tends to affect mostly women and MSM. The continued presence of bacteria in regional lymphatic channels leads to chronic inflammation and scarring, resulting in obstructive lymphedema, strictures, and fistulae formation. Ultimately, genital elephantiasis occurs,

known as *esthiomene* in women and *saxophone penis* in men.

In patients presenting primarily with proctitis or proctocolitis, the inguinal nodes do not drain the site of infection and are therefore not enlarged. However, deeper node involvement may lead to abdominal or pelvic discomfort. Initial symptoms consist of constipation or (less commonly) diarrhea along with a mucoid anorectal discharge. As the disease progresses, the anorectal discharge becomes bloody and tenesmus intensifies. As previously noted, nearly all cases of LGV recently diagnosed in industrialized countries have presented with signs and symptoms of proctocolitis rather than genital ulcers or inguinal lymphadenopathy.

Because of the low frequency of LGV, mass screening is not warranted. However, laboratory testing is indicated in those who present with proctitis and belong to a high-risk demographic group, present with inflammatory inguinal adenopathy and an appropriate travel history, or present with a history of sexual exposure to a known case of LGV.[55,58] Diseases most readily confused with LGV are those with prominent, painful adenopathy or lower gastrointestinal symptoms, including chancroid, herpes progenitalis, tuberculosis, cat scratch disease, plague and tularemia, lymphoma, irritable bowel syndrome, and inflammatory bowel diseases (Crohn's disease and ulcerative colitis).[58]

The precise diagnosis of LGV currently depends on identifying *C trachomatis*-specific DNA, followed by genotyping to verify known etiologic serovars L1, L2, or L3. The U.S. Food and Drug Administration has approved the use of nonspecific chlamydial nucleic acid amplification tests for genital swab and lymph node aspirate specimens, but these assays are not currently approved for use on rectal specimens. Nonetheless, they seem to be suitable screening tests when applied to specimens obtained from fresh anorectal discharge.

Several different molecular techniques are now available to confirm LGV-specific serovars in material that was found to be positive during screening for Chlamydia.[59,60] The CDC has recently announced that clinicians may send rectal swabs from patients whose symptoms suggest LGV to CDC laboratories to be tested with LGV-specific genotyping techniques that are not commercially available. Although direct culture would intuitively seem attractive, *C trachomatis* culture is difficult to perform and is available only in highly specialized laboratories.[61] A complement fixation serologic test to *C trachomatis* that is positive in a titer of more than 1:64 can support LGV diagnosis in the proper clinical context, but is neither as sensitive nor as specific as molecular testing.[61] In the absence of specific testing, the CDC also recommends that patients who have likely LGV based solely on clinical findings be treated for this presumptive diagnosis.

Treatment

Doxycycline is the preferred treatment of LGV and should be orally administered at a dosage of 100 mg twice daily for 21 days. Minocycline may also be used in a similar dosage schedule.[62] The actual evidence for using tetracycline derivatives in LGV is sparse and relies heavily on uncontrolled observations and clinical experience.[61] Alternatively, the CDC suggests that patients may receive erythromycin, 500 mg, orally four times daily for 21 days. High tissue concentration and a long half-life make azithromycin an attractive potential macrolide agent for treating LGV. However, minimal clinical data are available on the effectiveness of azithromycin for treating LGV.[63] No trials have been published on the use of fluoroquinolones in the management of LGV, and treatment failures have occurred after administration of sulfa drugs. Pregnant and lactating women should receive erythromycin rather than doxycycline. Although treatment cures infection, tissue scarring caused by chronic inflammation may not be reversible.

Other Treatment Considerations

Buboes may require needle aspiration or surgical drainage to achieve resolution. Patients diagnosed with LGV should be evaluated for other STDs, especially HIV. No comparative series indicate a higher failure rate of standard antibiotic therapy for LGV among those who are HIV coinfected; therefore, routine dosing schedules should be followed. Sexual contacts within 60 days of the index patient's symptom onset should be screened and perhaps treated with 1 week of doxycycline, 100 mg, twice daily.

GRANULOMA INGUINALE
Epidemiology

Similar to LGV, granuloma inguinale (GI) is a cause of GUD that infrequently occurs outside endemic areas, such as India, Southeast Asia, South Africa, the Caribbean basin, Brazil, Papua New Guinea, and aboriginal Australia. First described in 1882 in Madras, India, cases have been reported in industrialized countries, and clinicians should be aware of this disorder when constructing a differential diagnosis for GUD. Fewer than 10 cases are reported annually in the United States, and most are related to international travel. Men are infected two to six times more often than women, and infection rates peak in the third decade of life. In 1905, the Irish physician Charles Donovan described the presence of intracellular microorganisms in ulcer debris, and the disease was designated donovanosis in 1950 in honor of Dr. Donovan.[64] Both *donovanosis* and *granuloma inguinale* are considered proper terms for this infection.

The causative agent of GI is the intracellular gram-negative rod *Klebsiella granulomatis* (formerly known as *Donovania granulomatis* and *Calymmatobacterium granulomatis*). Although most cases of GI are clearly sexually transmitted, this may not be true in some instances. Evidence for this is summarized elsewhere and is beyond the scope of this manuscript.[64,65]

Clinical Presentation and Diagnosis

Most patients develop donovanosis within 6 weeks of exposure, although the incubation period may last 6 to 12 months. A reported case of experimental human inoculation yielded an incubation period of 50 days.[66] Single or multiple subcutaneous nodules develop at the inoculation site, and these nodules enlarge and erode, becoming surprisingly painless ulcers with clean bases and sharply demarcated, rolled margins. Ulcer bases are classically described as "beefy red" and consist of friable granulation tissue that bleeds readily when touched. Ulcers occur most commonly on the coronal sulcus in men and the labia minora in women.[67]

However, 6% of lesions are extragenital,[64] reportedly occurring on the lips and gums, oropharynx, nose, neck, and chest.[68] In the absence of bacterial superinfection, inguinal lymphadenopathy does not develop. Rather, subcutaneous edema and granulomas may lead to inguinal enlargement in approximately 10% of patients. These "pseudobuboes" may ulcerate or form abscesses, but this process is much less likely to occur in donovanosis compared with chancroid or LGV. Less commonly, lesions of GI may appear as hypertrophic or verrucous plaques, deeply necrotic ulcers, and cicatricial GI, (characterized by extensive tissue destruction followed by fibrosis and sclerosis).

Constitutional symptoms are not typically associated with GI, but severe local complications have been reported, including urethral and vaginal stenosis, and autoamputation of the penis. Untreated lesions have no tendency toward spontaneous resolution. Additionally, squamous cell carcinoma develops in 0.25% of cases and involvement of the cervix can lead to fatal hemorrhage during childbirth.

The differential diagnosis of GI includes other causes of genital ulcers, such as syphilis, chancroid, genital herpes, Behcet's syndrome, carcinoma, and cutaneous amebiasis. Because *K granulomatis* is difficult to isolate on any routine culture media,[69] GI is clinically diagnosed when visualizing Donovan bodies in a crush preparation of granulation tissue obtained from the ulcer base through scraping or punch biopsy and stained with Wright's, Giemsa, Warthin-Starry, or other stains that show fine cytologic detail. Ultrathin tissue samples are optimal for disclosing the characteristic Donovon bodies.[70] Donovan bodies appear as bipolar safety-pin shaped rods located within mononuclear cells and represent the actual infecting bacteria engulfed by macrophages and monocytes. Although molecular identification techniques have been developed,[71] these are not readily available, even in local and state health laboratories.

Treatment

Few studies have been conducted to determine optimal treatment for GI, but the traditionally preferred treatment is with doxycycline (100 mg orally twice daily for at least 3 weeks or until lesions have healed). However, using any tetracycline derivatives to manage GI now has a relatively high risk for therapeutic failure worldwide.[67] Alternative medications include trimethoprim-sulfamethoxazole (one 160 mg/800 mg tablet orally twice daily), ciprofloxacin (750 mg orally twice daily), erythromycin (500 mg orally four times daily), or azithromycin (1 g orally once weekly). In Australia, azithromycin has also been dosed at 500 mg daily for 1 week (or until lesions have healed).[72] Aminoglycosides, such as gentamicin (1 mg/kg three times daily, intramuscularly), may also be efficacious but are not considered first-line agents because of potential toxicity. Ceftriaxone (1 g daily, intramuscularly) has had only limited published use.[73] trimethoprim-sulfamethoxazole is probably the best alternative to doxycycline and may actually be the preferred drug for current American cases.[67] Treatment with these various regimens should continue for at least 3 weeks or until all lesions clinically heal. Surgical intervention may be necessary to repair extensive tissue destruction in advanced cases.[74]

Other Treatment Considerations

As with the other causes of GUD, patients diagnosed with GI should be screened for additional STDs and HIV. All treatments are continued until clinical cure, and therefore HIV coinfection does not seem to affect therapeutic interventions.

Because fluoroquinolones, tetracycline derivatives, and sulfa drugs are either absolutely or relatively contraindicated in pregnancy, erythromycin and azithromycin regimens are preferred during gestation despite the lack of adequate studies.[20]

GONORRHEA
Epidemiology

Gonorrhea, caused by the gram-negative intracellular diplococcus *Neisseria gonorrhoeae*, has been a common human pathogen since the disease was named by the Greek physician, Galen, in the second century. However, not until the late 19th century were gonorrhea and syphilis recognized as two different diseases, and Albert Neisser first identified the gonococcus after examining the purulent urethral exudates. The worldwide incidence is estimated at least to be 60 million cases annually, with more than 300,000 new cases occurring each year in the United States alone. In 2006, 358,366 cases of gonorrhea were reported in the United States, equivalent to a rate of 120.9 cases per 100,000 population.[14] This represented an increase of 5.5% since 2005 and an increased rate for the second consecutive year. The disease is especially prevalent in African Americans, Hispanic adolescents, prison inmates, commercial sex workers, MSM, and patients who have HIV. Up to 15% of MSM tested have evidence of gonorrheal infections, with the pharynx the most common site. A great many of these are asymptomatic and would be missed without selective screening tests for high-risk groups.[75,76]

Clinical Presentation and Diagnosis

Although most cases of gonorrhea produce signs and symptoms restricted to the urogenital tract, prominent cutaneous manifestations may develop in local infection sites (eg, Bartholin's or Skene's glands) or when the infection disseminates. After a short incubation period (1 day to 2 weeks), patients infected with *N gonorrhoeae* may develop signs and symptoms of inflammation at the primary inoculation site. Common presenting complaints include pharyngitis; urethritis; intense burning or painful dysuria; profuse, purulent urethral discharge; and pelvic pain. However, up to one half of patients will have completely asymptomatic infections. Rarely, primary cutaneous lesions develop.

If the inoculation is from sexual contact or traumatic inoculation, genital pustules or a morphologically typical furuncle may appear.[77,78] The most prominent cutaneous manifestations occur when the gonococcal infection disseminates widely. Disseminated gonoccocal infection (DGI) develops in 1% to 3% of cases and usually occurs in young, otherwise healthy patients who have asymptomatic genital, rectal, or oropharyngeal infection.[79] Other risk factors for DGI development include hereditary defects in the terminal complement pathway and persistent hypocomplementemia (eg, caused by lupus erythematosus). Two distinct clinical presentations exist and may occur concomitantly in cases of DGI. The *septic arthritis syndrome* is characterized as a febrile illness associated with inflammation affecting one or more joints (inflammation manifesting as pain, swelling, erythema, and decreased range of motion).

The more common *tenosynovitis-arthritis-dermatitis syndrome* occurs in 60% of cases of DGI. Patients develop tender erythema over tendons and tendinous bony insertion sites. Additionally, a migratory, pauciarticular arthralgia or arthritis occurs, involving appendicular joints. Typically, fewer than three joints are affected. The characteristic skin lesions of DGI begin as nonspecific erythematous macules that quickly progress to form tender necrotic pustules or hemorrhagic bullae. These skin lesions appear on the dorsal aspect of distal extremities near the joints of the wrists, hands, and ankles. Pustules result from bacterial embolization, followed by microabscess formation. Characteristically, very few lesions are present.

In symptomatic men, a Gram stain of the urethral discharge is virtually always positive and diagnostic of gonorrhea. However, Gram stains of oropharyngeal, rectal, or endocervical specimens lack the appropriate sensitivity and specificity for diagnosis. In cases of DGI, cultures of blood or specimens obtained directly from cutaneous lesions rarely yield positive results. Gene amplification techniques are recommended for diagnosis in these cases. Therefore, DGI should be diagnosed based on clinical findings and isolation of *N gonorrhoeae* from the primary site of infection. Culture of *N gonorrhoeae* offers the added benefit of determining antimicrobial susceptibility and allowing for appropriate therapy.

Treatment

Because of the ongoing evolution of drug resistance in wild strains of *N gonorrhoeae*, the CDC makes frequent updates to its recommendations for gonorrhea therapy. Currently, only cephalosporins are recommended as first-line therapy; because of high levels of fluoroquinolone resistance, these drugs were recently eliminated from the treatment algorithm. Patients who have uncomplicated infections of the urethra, rectum, or cervix may be treated with ceftriaxone (125 mg,

intramuscularly, in a single dose) or cefixime (400 mg, orally, in a single dose).[80] Patients allergic to cephalosporin should be treated with spectinomycin (2 g, intramuscularly, as a single dose). Azithromycin in a single 2.0-g dose is also effective for uncomplicated gonococcal infection but is not recommended because of frequent gastrointestinal distress at that dosage level.[80]

Management of DGI requires more aggressive intervention, and patients generally should be hospitalized initially so they can be carefully monitored for complications, such as bacterial endocarditis, meningitis, or perihepatitis. Parenteral antibiotics are indicated in DGI. The recommended regimen is with ceftriaxone (1 g, intramuscularly or intravenous, every 24 hours), with alternatives including cefotaxime (1 g, intravenously, every 8 hours) and ceftizoxime (1 g, every 8 hours).[80] Treatment with intravenous antibiotics should continue for 24 to 48 hours after clinical improvement begins, and then patients may be switched to cefotaxime (400 mg, orally, twice daily) for a minimum total of one week of antibiotic therapy. Patients with known cephalosporin allergy should receive spectinomycin (2 g intramuscularly every 12 hours) for the same total duration.

Other Treatment Considerations

Patients diagnosed with gonorrhea should be evaluated for other STDs, including syphilis and HIV. Because patients infected with gonorrhea are often coinfected with *C trachomatis*, nonspecific chlamydial nucleic acid amplification tests (NAATs) should routinely be performed on patients who have gonorrhea. Because of the high sensitivity of NAATs for chlamydial infection, a negative test eliminates the need for concomitant therapy. However, if chlamydial tests are not performed or the results are unavailable, then patients should be simultaneously treated for both gonorrhea and chlamydia. The latter can be accomplished by administering a single oral 1.0-g dose of azithromycin or a 1-week course of doxycycline (100 mg, twice daily).[80]

GENITAL BITE WOUNDS

Genital bite wounds are most likely underreported and underdiagnosed. Patients who have genital bite wounds often seek medical care late in the course of disease because of embarrassment and protracted attempts at self-treatment.[81] This subject receives little attention in the medical literature, and therefore clinicians have few updated diagnostic or therapeutic recommendations.

Traumatic orogenital contact occurs frequently and results from sexual practices or intentional attempt at harm. The exact incidence of genital bite wounds is unknown. The clinical presentation of a patient who has a genital bite wound depends on the time that has elapsed since the injury and the severity of the etiologic trauma. Patients may present with notably painful, superficially to deeply necrotic lacerations or ulcerations of the external genitalia, which literally develop in just 1 to several days after the traumatic event.[82,83]

Although most genital wounds are superficial, the loose subcutaneous tissue of the perineum facilitates the spread of microorganisms and creates the potential for severe complications, including rapidly advancing cellulitis, balanoposthitis, Fournier's gangrene, abscess formation, lymphangitis, and even sepsis.[81] The most important complication of genital bite wounds is the risk for infection with human oropharyngeal flora. Although infections are nearly always polymicrobial, they most commonly involve the human oral flora microbe *Eikenella corrodens*.[82–84] Particularly aggressive orogenital contact can also result in disfigurement and may ultimately lead to sexual dysfunction, urethral strictures, and fistulae formation. Additionally, transmission of diseases such as syphilis, viral hepatitis, tetanus, tuberculosis, and HIV has been reported to occur, albeit rarely, through human bites.

Wounds should be cultured for aerobic and anaerobic bacteria, and additional assessment with Darkfield microscopy and viral culture may be warranted. Wounds that follow traumatic orogenital events should be cleansed with copious irrigation using a bactericidal and virucidal solution, such as 1% povidone-iodine. Because of the high risk for infection, genital wounds accompanying a bite should never be closed primarily.

The medical literature contains no standardized or evidence-based recommendations for treatment of genital bite wounds. However, empiric antibiotic therapy should cover for potential pathogens, such as gram-positive cocci and gram-negative rods, especially *E corrodens*. Successful treatment has been reported with amoxicillin-clavulanic acid (500 mg/125 mg, twice daily for 14 days).[82,83] Alternatives may include second-generation cephalosporins (eg, cefuroxime) or combination therapy with dicloxacillin and penicillin.[84] Antibiotic therapy should ultimately be adjusted according to antimicrobial sensitivity results obtained from wound cultures whenever feasible.

REFERENCES

1. De Schryver A, Meheus A. Epidemiology of sexually transmitted diseases: the global picture. Bull World Health Organ 1990;68(5):639–54.

2. Da Ros CT, Schmitt Cda S. Global epidemiology of sexually transmitted diseases. Asian J Androl 2008; 10(1):110–4.

3. World Health Organization. Sexually transmitted infections fact sheet. Available at: http://www.who.int/mediacentre/factsheets/fs110/en/index.html. Accessed October, 2007.

4. Wasserheit JN. Epidemiologic synergy. Interrelationships between human immunodeficiency virus infection and other sexually transmitted diseases. Sex Transm Dis 1992;19(2):61–77.

5. Dickerson MC, Johnston J, Delea TE, et al. The causal role for genital ulcer disease as a risk factor for transmission of human immunodeficiency virus. An application of the Bradford Hill criteria. Sex Transm Dis 1996;23(5):429–40.

6. Fleming DT, Wasserheit JN. From epidemiological synergy to public health policy and practice: the contribution of other sexually transmitted diseases to sexual transmission of HIV infection. Sex Transm Infect 1999;75(1):3–17.

7. Risbud A. Human immunodeficiency virus (HIV) and sexually transmitted diseases (STD). Indian J Med Res 2005;121(4):369–76.

8. Grosskurth H, Mosha F, Todd J, et al. Impact of improved treatment of sexually transmitted diseases on HIV infection in rural Tanzania: randomized controlled trial. Lancet 1995;346(8974):530–6.

9. Kamali A, Quigley M, Nakiyingi J, et al. Syndromic management of sexually transmitted infections and behaviour change interventions on transmission of HIV-1 in rural Uganda: a community randomized trial. Lancet 2003;361(9358):645–52.

10. Laxminarayan R, Mills AJ, Breman JG, et al. Advancement of global health: key messages from the disease control priorities project. Lancet 2006; 367(9517):1193–208.

11. Centers for Disease Control and Prevention. Trends in reportable sexually transmitted diseases in the United States, 2004-national surveillance data for chlamydia, gonorrhea, and syphilis. Atlanta (GA): U.S. Department of Health and Human Services (National Center for HIV, STD, and TB Prevention); 2004.

12. Rothschild BM. History of syphilis. Clin Infect Dis 2005;40(10):1454–63.

13. Rompalo AM. Can syphilis be eradicated from the world? Curr Opin Infect Dis 2001;14(1):41–4.

14. Centers for Disease Control and Prevention. Sexually transmitted disease surveillance, 2006. Atlanta (GA): U.S. Department of Health and Human Services (National Center for HIV, STD, and TB Prevention); 2007.

15. Peterman TA, Furness BW. The resurgence of syphilis among men who have sex with men. Curr Opin Infect Dis 2007;20(1):54–9.

16. Centers for Disease Control and Prevention. The national plan to eliminate syphilis from the United

States. Atlanta (GA): U.S. Department of Health and Human Services (National Center for HIV, STD, and TB Prevention); 2006.

17. Golden MR, Marra CM, Holmes KK. Update on syphilis: resurgence of an old problem. JAMA 2003;290(11):1510–4.

18. Hutchinson CM, Hook EW 3rd, Shepherd M, et al. Altered clinical presentation of early syphilis in patients with human immunodeficiency virus infection. Ann Intern Med 1994;121(2):94–100.

19. Zeltser R, Kurban AK. Syphilis. Clin Dermatol 2004; 22(6):461–8.

20. Centers for Disease Control and Prevention. Sexually transmitted diseases treatment guidelines, 2006. MMWR Morb Mortal Wkly Rep 2006;55(No. RR-11): 1–94.

21. Verdon MS, Handsfield HH, Johnson RB. Pilot study of azithromycin for treatment of primary and secondary syphilis. Clin Infect Dis 1994;19(3):486–8.

22. Gruber F, Kastelan M, Cabrijan L, et al. Treatment of early syphilis with azithromycin. J Chemother 2000; 12(3):240–3.

23. Hook EW III, Martin DH, Stephens J, et al. A randomized, comparative pilot study of azithromycin versus benzathine penicillin G for treatment of early syphilis. Sex Transm Dis 2002;29(8):486–90.

24. Riedner G, Rusizoka M, Todd J, et al. Single-dose azithromycin versus penicillin G benzathine for the treatment of early syphilis. N Engl J Med 2005; 353(12):1236–44.

25. Kiddugavu MG, Kiwanuka N, Wawer MJ, et al. Effectiveness of syphilis treatment using azithromycin and/or benzathine penicillin in Rakai, Uganda. Sex Transm Dis 2005;32(1):1–6.

26. Centers for Disease Control and Prevention. Azithromycin treatment failures in syphilis infections—San Francisco, California, 2002–2003. MMWR Morb Mortal Wkly Rep 2004;53(9):197–8.

27. Lukehart SA, Godornes C, Molini BJ, et al. Macrolide resistance in Treponema pallidum in the United States and Ireland. N Engl J Med 2004;351(2):154–8.

28. Katz KA, Klausner JD. Azithromycin resistance in Treponema pallidum. Curr Opin Infect Dis 2008; 21(1):83–91.

29. Moorthy TT, Lee CT, Lim KB, et al. Ceftriaxone for treatment of primary syphilis in men: a preliminary study. Sex Transm Dis 1987;14(2):116–8.

30. Zhou P, Gu Z, Xu J, et al. A study evaluating ceftriaxone as a treatment agent for primary and secondary syphilis in pregnancy. Sex Transm Dis 2005;32(8):495–8.

31. Augenbraun M, Workowski K. Ceftriaxone therapy for syphilis: report from the emerging infections network. Clin Infect Dis 1999;29(5):1337–8.

32. Smith NH, Musher DM, Huang DB, et al. Response of HIV-infected patients with asymptomatic syphilis to intensive intramuscular therapy with ceftriaxone or procaine penicillin. Int J STD AIDS 2004;15(5):328–32.

33. Rolfs RT, Joesoef MR, Hendershot EF, et al. A randomized trial of enhanced therapy for early syphilis in patients with and without human immunodeficiency virus infection. The Syphilis and HIV Study Group. N Engl J Med 1997;337(5):307–14.

34. Bong CT, Bauer ME, Spinola SM. Haemophilus ducreyi: clinical features, epidemiology, and prospects for disease control. Microbes Infect 2002;4(11):1141–8.

35. Sehgal VN, Srivastava G. Chancroid: contemporary appraisal. Int J Dermatol 2003;42(3):182–90.

36. Jones C, Rosen T, Clarridge J, et al. Chancroid: results from an outbreak in Houston, Texas. South Med J 1990;83(12):1384–9.

37. Lewis DA. Chancroid: clinical manifestations, diagnosis, and management. Sex Transm Infect 2003; 79(1):68–71.

38. Brown TJ, Yen-Moore A, Tyring SK. An overview of sexually transmitted diseases. Part I. J Am Acad Dermatol 1999;41(4):511–32.

39. Smith JL, Bayles DO. The contribution of cytolethal distending toxin to bacterial pathogenesis. Crit Rev Microbiol 2006;32(4):227–48.

40. Jones CC, Rosen T. Cultural diagnosis of chancroid. Arch Dermatol 1991;127(12):1823–7.

41. Patterson K, Olsen B, Thomas C, et al. Development of a rapid immunodiagnostic test for Haemophilus ducreyi. J Clin Microbiol 2002;40(10):3694–702.

42. Tyndall M, Malisa M, Plummer FA, et al. Ceftriaxone no longer predictably cures chancroid in Kenya. J Infect Dis 1993;167(2):469–71.

43. Tyndall MW, Agoki E, Plummer FA, et al. Single dose azithromycin for the treatment of chancroid: a randomized comparison with erythromycin. Sex Transm Dis 1994;21(4):231–4.

44. Roy-Leon JE, Lauzon WD, Toye B, et al. In vitro and in vivo activity of combination antimicrobial agents on Haemophilus ducreyi. J Antimicrob Chemother 2005;56(3):552–8.

45. Afonina G, Leduc I, Nepluev I, et al. Immunization with the Haemophilus ducreyi hemoglobin receptor HgbA protects against infection in the swine model of chancroid. Infect Immun 2006;74(4):2224–32.

46. Nieuwenhuis RF, Ossewaarde JM, van der Meijden WI, et al. Unusual presentation of early lymphogranuloma venereum in an HIV-1 infected patient: effective treatment with 1 g azithromycin. Sex Transm Infect 2003;79(6):453–5.

47. Van de Laar MJ, Gotz H, de Zwart O, et al. Lymphogranuloma venereum among men who have sex with men—Netherlands, 2003–2004. MMWR Morb Mortal Wkly Rep 2004;53(42):985–8.

48. Nieuwenhuis RF, Ossewaarde JM, Gotz HM, et al. Resurgence of lymphogranuloma venereum in Western Europe: an outbreak of Chlamydia trachomatis serovar L2 proctitis in The Netherlands among men who have sex with men. Clin Infect Dis 2004; 39(7):996–1003.

49. Herida M, de Barbeyrac B, Sednaoui P, et al. Rectal lymphogranuloma venereum surveillance in France 2004–2005. Euro Surveill 2006;11(9):155–6.

50. Meyer T, Arndt R, von Krosigk A, et al. Repeated detection of lymphogranuloma venereum caused by Chlamydia trachomatis L2 in homosexual men in Hamburg. Sex Transm Infect 2005;81(1):91–2.

51. Kropp RY, Wong T. Emergence of Lymphogranuloma venereum in Canada. CMAJ 2005;172(13):1674–6.

52. Ahdoot A, Kotler DP, Suh JS, et al. Lymphogranuloma venereum in human immunodeficiency virus-infected individuals in New York City. J Clin Gastroenterol 2006;40(5):385–90.

53. Ward H, Martin I, Macdonald N, et al. Lymphogranuloma venereum in the United kingdom. Clin Infect Dis 2007;44(1):26–32.

54. van de Laar MJ. The emergence of LGV in Western Europe: what do we know, what can we do? Euro Surveill 2006;11(9):146–8.

55. de Vries HJ, Fennema JS, Morre SA. Lymphogranuloma venereum among men having sex with men; what have we learned so far? Sex Transm Infect 2006;82(4):344.

56. Spaargaren J, Schachter J, Moncada J, et al. Slow epidemic of lymphogranuloma venereum L2b strain. Emerg Infect Dis 2005;11(11):1787–8.

57. Buntin DM, Rosen T, Lesher JL Jr, et al. Sexually transmitted diseases: bacterial infections. J Am Acad Dermatol 1991;25:287–99.

58. Herring A, Richens J. Lymphogranuloma venereum. Sex Transm Infect 2006;82(Suppl 4):iv23–25.

59. Sturm PD, Moodley P, Govender K, et al. Molecular diagnosis of lymphogranuloma venereum in patients with genital ulcer disease. J Clin Microbiol 2005;43(6):2973–5.

60. Morre S, Spaargaren J, Fennema JS, et al. Molecular diagnosis of lymphogranuloma venereum: PCR-based restriction fragment length polymorphism and real-time PCR. J Clin Microbiol 2005;43(10):5412–3.

61. McLean CA, Stoner BP, Workowski KA. Treatment of lymphogranuloma venereum. Clin Infect Dis 2007;44(Suppl 3):S147–152.

62. Sowmini CN, Gopalan KN, Rao GC. Minocycline in the treatment of lymphogranuloma venereum. J Am Vener Dis Assoc 1976;2:19–22.

63. Ballard RC, Ye H, Matta A, et al. Treatment of chancroid with azithromycin. Int J STD AIDS 1996;7:9–12.

64. O'Farrell N. Donovanosis. Sex Transm Infect 2002;78(6):452–7.

65. Lupi O, Madkan V, Tyring SK. Tropical dermatology: bacterial tropical diseases. J Am Acad Dermatol 2006;54(4):559–78.

66. Greenblatt RB, Dient RB, Torpin R. Experimental and clinical granuloma inguinale. JAMA 1939;113(11):1109–16.

67. Rosen T, Tchen JA, Ramsdell W, et al. Granuloma inguinale. J Am Acad Dermatol 1984;11(3):433–7.

68. Hart G. Donovanosis. Clin Infect Dis 1997;25(1):24–30.

69. Brennand GLP, Santana EM, Jardim ML. Cultivation of Calymmatobacterium granulomatis in mouse peritoneal macrophage monolayer. An Bras Dermatol 1999;74(3):357–8.

70. Joseph AK, Rosen T. Laboratory techniques used in the diagnosis of chancroid, granuloma inguinale, and lymphogranuloma. Dermatol Clin. 1994;12(1):1–8.

71. Bastian I, Bowden FJ. Amplification of Klebsiella-like sequences from biopsy samples from patients with donovanosis. Clin Infect Dis 1996;23(6):1328–30.

72. Bowden FJ, Mein J, Plunkett C, et al. Pilot study of azithromycin in the treatment of genital donovanosis. Genitourin Med 1994;72(1):17–9.

73. Merianos A, Gilles M, Chuah J. Ceftriaxone in the treatment of chronic donovanosis in central Australia. Genitourin Med 1994;70(2):84–9.

74. Parkash S, Radhakrishna K. Problemic ulcerative lesions in sexually transmitted diseases: surgical management. Sex Transm Dis 1986;13(3):127–33.

75. Morris SR, Klausner JD, Buchbinder SP, et al. Prevalence and incidence of pharyngeal gonorrhea in a longitudinal sample of men who have sex with men: the EXPLORE study. Clin Infect Dis 2006;43(10):1284–9.

76. Kent CK, Chaw JK, Wong W, et al. Prevalence of rectal, urethral, and pharyngeal chlamydia and gonorrhea detected in 2 clinical settings among men who have sex with men: San Francisco, California, 2003. Clin Infect Dis 2005;41(1):67–74.

77. Rosen T. Unusual presentations of gonorrhea. J Am Acad Dermatol 1982;6(3):369–72.

78. Ghosn SH, Kibbi AG. Cutaneous gonococcal infections. Clin Dermatol 2004;22(6):476–80.

79. Mehrany K, Kist JM, O'Connor WJ, et al. Disseminated gonococcemia. Int J Dermatol 2003;42(3):208–9.

80. Centers for Disease Control and Prevention. Updated recommended treatment regimens for gonococcal infections and associated conditions. Atlanta (GA): U.S. Department of Health and Human Services (National Center for HIV, STD, and TB Prevention); 2007. Available at: http://www.cdc.gov/std/treatment/2006/updated-regimens.htm. Accessed March 2, 2008.

81. Wolf JS Jr, Gomez R, McAninch JW. Human bites to the penis. J Urol 1992;147(5):1265–7.

82. Rosen T, Conrad N. Genital ulcer caused by human bite to the penis. Sex Transm Dis 1999;26(9):527–30.

83. Rosen T. Penile ulcer from traumatic orogenital contact. Dermatol Online J 2005;11(2):18.

84. Griego RD, Rosen T, Orengo IF, et al. Dog, cat, and human bites: a review. J Am Acad Dermatol 1995;33(6):1019–29.

Atypical Mycobacterial Cutaneous Infections

Sanjay Bhambri, DO[a],*, Avani Bhambri, MD[b],
James Q. Del Rosso, DO, FAOCD[a]

KEYWORDS

- Atypical mycobacteria • Nontuberculous • Mycobacteria
- *M. marinum* • *M. avium-intracellulare* • *M. kansasii*
- *M. simiae* • *M. ulceran*

Mycobacterium tuberculosis and *M leprae* are widely known to cause many infections worldwide. Atypical mycobacterial infection is a term applied to infections caused by mycobacteria other than *M tuberculosis* and *M leprae*. Mycobacteria other than typical tubercle and leprae bacilli or nontuberculous mycobacteria (NTM) were originally known as atypical, tuberculoid, opportunistic, or anonymous mycobacteria.[1] NTM have been a cause of steadily growing infections over the past decades, especially in patients who have compromised immune status. NTM are slender, nonmotile, non–spore forming acid-fast bacilli.

Atypical mycobacteria are found in many environmental areas, such as wet soil, house dust, water, dairy products, cold-blooded animals, vegetation, and human feces. The bacteria are accidentally transmitted by inhalation, ingestion, or percutaneous penetration and can cause disease in the skin, lungs, lymph nodes, and skeletal and genitourinary systems.[2]

The development of disease depends on many factors, such as mycobacterium species, the degree of exposure, and the immune status of the host. Delayed diagnosis is common and is often attributable to lack of clinical suspicion. It is not easy to identify the NTM by culture or the traditional histochemical Ziehl-Neelsen stain. Polymerase chain reaction (PCR) may be necessary to identify the organism. The most common NTM causing human disease in the United States is *M avium-intracellulare* (MAI).[2]

CLASSIFICATION

The genus mycobacterium is divided into obligate and facultative pathogens. The obligate group involves *M tuberculosis* and *M leprae*. The facultative group is divided into slow-growing and rapid-growing mycobacteria. Runyon further classified the slow-growing mycobacteria based on their ability to produce pigment, growth rate, and optimal temperature.[3,4] This classification is depicted in **Table 1**.

Photochromogens produce pigment only when exposed to light. Scotochromogens produce pigment under both light and dark conditions. Nonchromogens do not produce pigment. Group IV mycobacteria are rapid growers because of their unique ability to display mature colonies rapidly.

GROUP I: PHOTOCHROMOGENS
Mycobacterium Marinum (*Mycobacterium Balnei* or *Mycobacterium Platypoecilus*)

M marinum is a slow-growing photochromogen that usually causes disease in fish but can cause human disease by penetration through impaired skin barrier. It was first discovered in 1926 by Aronson who isolated the organism from a saltwater fish in a Philadelphia aquarium.[5] The first human case was reported in 1951 in a patient who developed granulomatous lesions after visiting a contaminated swimming pool.[6] The disease caused by *M marinum* is sometimes referred to

[a] Valley Hospital Medical Center, Medical Education Department, 620 Shadow Lane, Las Vegas, NV 89106, USA
[b] University of California Los Angeles Medical Center, Los Angeles, CA 90095, USA
* Corresponding author.
E-mail address: sbhambri18@hotmail.com (S. Bhambri).

Dermatol Clin 27 (2009) 63–73
doi:10.1016/j.det.2008.07.009
0733-8635/08/$ – see front matter © 2009 Published by Elsevier Inc.

Table 1
Classification of atypical mycobacteria

Group I	Photochromogens	Yellow pigment	M.marinum M.kansasii M.simiae
Group II	Scotochromogens	Yellow-orange pigment	M.scrofulaceum M.szulgai
Group III	Nonchromogens		M.avium-intracellulare M.ulcerans M.haemophilum
Group IV	Rapid growing		M.fortuitum M.chelonei M.abscessus

as swimming pool granuloma or fish tank granuloma.

M marinum is normally found in salt water, fresh water, or brackish water sources, such as swimming pools, rivers, lakes, oceans, and aquariums. Many vectors have been identified, including shrimp, dolphins, snails, water fleas, and saltwater and freshwater fish.[1,7–9] Traumas, such as abrasions and puncture wounds, seem to play a role in the occurrence of the disease. Other risk factors, such as occupation or hobbies involving a fish-related job or home aquarium, have also been implicated.[10] Dodiuk-Gad and colleagues[10] conducted a retrospective study of 25 patients who had NTM infections of the skin. *M marinum* was found to be the organism responsible for disease in 16 out of 25 patients. Some 75% of patients either had a fish-related job or had reared fish in a home aquarium.

M marinum is an aerobic organism that grows at a temperature of 30°C to 32°C on Lowenstein-Jensen medium in 2 to 5 weeks. The organism grows poorly or is absent at 37°C. The color changes from white to yellow-orange when exposed to light.[11] The organism tests negative for nitrate reductase and niacin but positive for catalase.[10,12]

Ho and colleagues[2,9,13,14] conducted a 10-year retrospective study of NTM infections in Hong Kong. *M marinum* was the most common organism, responsible for disease in more than 50% of patients. The culture positivity for *M marinum* was 76.5%, whereas the overall culture-positive rate was 54.5%, thereby suggesting that a culture is specific but not sensitive.

Anti–tumor necrosis factor (TNF)–α therapy is increasingly being used to treat patients who have diseases such as psoriasis, psoriatic arthritis, rheumatoid arthritis, and Crohn disease. There are three TNF-α inhibitors available in the market today: etanercept, adalimumab, and infliximab.

M marinum infection associated with TNF-α inhibitors was first reported in 1994 in a patient who developed septic arthritis associated with etanercept therapy.[15] Similar infections have been reported with both etanercept and infliximab.[16–19]

Clinical features

Lesions are usually localized at the site of the inoculation with a predilection for areas predisposed to trauma.[20,21] The most common area of involvement is the extremities with the finger being the most common site (**Fig. 1**), and thus the infection is referred to as "fish tank finger."[10,21,22] Because exposure to contaminated water is important in the development of lesions, it is not surprising to see disease on the backs of hands of fish handlers and on the feet, elbows, and knees of swimmers.

Lesions can appear in a superficial (type I), granulomatous (type II), or deep (type III) pattern after an incubation period of 2 to 8 weeks.[21,23] Superficial lesions are self-limited and usually appear as a bluish-red erythematous papule or pustule that

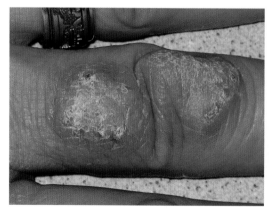

Fig. 1. Erythematous nodules located on the dorsal aspect of finger. "Fish tank finger" caused by *M marinum*.

may increase in size to form a verrucous or violaceous plaque or nodule.[1,20,24,25] Superficial lesions are usually solitary and frequently undergo central ulceration. Type II lesions present as solitary or multiple granulomas, with or without ulceration. The most common reported symptom is pain, with others being tenderness, swelling, drainage, and pruritus.

Disseminated lesions or deep infections involving tendons, bones, joints, and bursae have been reported in immunocompromised patients, such as in renal transplant recipients, patients who have systemic lupus erythematosus, and those on chronic steroid therapy.[26–28] Deeper infections can lead to tenosynovitis, osteomyelitis, bone erosions, and bursitis.[21]

A sporotrichoid distribution with lesions along sites of lymphatic drainage has also been seen with M marinum, especially in immunocompromised patients.[1,7,10,11,25] Infection with the organism does not lead to immunity and thus reinfection with M marinum is possible.[11]

Histopathology

The pathology findings are variable and depend on how long the lesion has been present. Biopsy must be taken from a non-ulcerated area that is in close proximity to the lesion.[21] A nonspecific inflammation, consisting of a mixed infiltrate including lymphocytes, neutrophils, and histiocytes, is seen.[1] Granulomatous inflammatory infiltrate mimicking tuberculoid granuloma, sarcoid-like granuloma, or rheumatoid-like nodules may be noted.[4,21] In chronic (after 6 months) lesions, a tuberculoid granuloma with fibrinoid necrosis without true caseation was noted.[1]

Travis and colleagues[22] reported a histopathologic spectrum of M marinum infection. Epidermal changes included pseudoepitheliomatous hyperplasia, acanthosis, focal parakeratosis, and follicular plugging. Poorly formed granulomas were noted in 4 of 5 patients and consisted of collections of epithelioid histiocytes and lymphocytes with low multinucleated giant cells. Abscess formation varied from absent (2 of 5) to moderate (2 of 5) to marked (1 of 5). Kullavanijaya and colleagues noted a mononuclear cell granuloma in biopsies of 16 out of 18 patients who had lesions attributable to M marinum.[29] PCR-ELISA can be beneficial in identifying the organism.[30–35]

Treatment

No specific criteria exist for the treatment of infections caused by NTM. Several modalities have been reported as effective and they include spontaneous resolution, surgery, cryotherapy, electrode therapy, and irradiation. Spontaneous resolution in 24 to 36 months has been described.[1] Deeper infections, such as tenosynovitis, do not heal and can cause significant impairment if not treated.[21] Surgical treatment may be necessary for deeper lesions to remove the necrotic tissue and should be combined with medications to ensure proper treatment.

Antibiotics are the mainstay of therapy; however, treatment failures have been reported with all antibiotics. The tetracycline family of antibiotics, including minocycline and doxycycline, are effective in treating M marinum infections. M marinum was also shown to be sensitive to some antituberculous drugs, such as rifampicin and ethambutol, while being resistant to others, such as isoniazid and streptomycin.[26]

A multidrug approach is often used to minimize the risk for resistance. Dodiuk-Gad and colleagues[10] noted 100% sensitivity of M marinum to clarithromycin, streptomycin, and ethionamide, but revealed resistance of some strains to quinolones. A treatment regimen, including clarithromycin 500 mg twice a day, rifampin 600 mg daily, and ethambutol 25 mg/kg daily, has been shown to be effective.[1]

Co-trimoxazole was reported to be effective in clearing lesions in 1 to 6 months.[25,29] Monotherapy with minocycline or doxycycline 100 mg twice daily has been reported to be successful with complete clearance of lesions in 3 months.[26] Patients should be treated for a period of 3 to 6 months with at least 4 to 8 weeks of therapy after the resolution of lesions.

Rallis and colleagues[18] reported a case of sporotrichoid M marinum infection associated with infliximab. Lesions resolved with a combination of rifampin 600 mg daily and ethambutol 15 to 25 mg/kg/d despite continuation of infliximab, thereby suggesting that discontinuation of anti–TNF-α therapy is not necessary. More data are needed to confirm or validate these findings.

Mycobacterium Kansasii

M kansasii is a slow-growing photochromogen that primarily affects lung tissue.[12,29] The organism is usually seen in cattle and swine but has also been isolated from tap water and ice machines.[12] The organism can stay in water for as long as 12 months.[36] It grows at 37°C on Lowenstein-Jensen, Middlebrook 7H10 media and BACTEC 128 broth and produces yellow pigment after exposure to light. The organism is niacin negative but displays strong catalase reaction.[7] It has been reported that infection with this organism provides increased immunity against tuberculosis.[7]

Clinical features

M kansasii usually affects diseased lung tissue, such as patients who have chronic obstructive pulmonary disease (COPD) and cystic fibrosis.[7,12] Patients often have a history of immunosuppression or trauma. Cutaneous lesions are usually composed of papules and pustules often forming verrucous or granulomatous plaques or nodules that may ulcerate. A sporotrichoid pattern or cellulitis has also been noted as a presenting feature.[36]

Histopathology

A granulomatous histology and a mixed inflammatory infiltrate, with acid-fast bacilli in the histiocytes, are usually noted. Chronic tuberculoid granulomas are devoid of organisms. Histopathology is identical to tuberculosis and thus the diagnosis must be confirmed by isolation and identification of the organism. Epidermal necrosis and abscess formation may be noted on histology. Perivascular mononuclear infiltration without granuloma formation may be noted.[36] Culture of the biopsied specimen and PCR-ELISA can be beneficial in identifying the organism.[37]

Treatment

Treatment regimen of isoniazid 300 to 600 mg daily, rifampin 600 mg daily, and ethambutol 15 mg/kg daily for 18 to 24 months has been shown to be effective.[7,12,38–40] Streptomycin 1 g intramuscularly (IM) twice weekly can be added to the regimen for the first 3 months, especially in patients who have AIDS. Resistance to kanamycin and trimethoprim-sulfamethoxazole has been reported.[41,42] Surgical débridement of the lesions combined with oral ethambutol, cycloserine, and rifampin for 1 year has also been reported to be effective.[41]

Mycobacterium Simiae

M simiae complex is composed of several species, including M simiae, M triplex, M genavense, M heidelbergense, and M lentiflavum. M simiae was first isolated by Karasseva and Krasznay from rhesus monkeys in 1965.[43–45] M simiae is an opportunistic acid-fast bacillus that usually causes infection in immunocompromised hosts. It is a slow-growing photochromogen that changes to a rust color after exposure to light. The organism can be cultured on Lowenstein-Jensen or Middlebrook media in less than 6 weeks and is the only niacin-positive NTM. It is normally found in the southwestern United States (Arizona, New Mexico, Texas), Cuba, and Israel.[43–45] M simiae outbreak has been associated with hospital water supply in one instance.[45]

Clinical features

Lymphadenitis has been seen in immunocompetent and immunocompromised patients. Persistent fever and debilitation without localizing signs were the most common clinical features in disseminated M simiae infection.[46]

Histopathology

Necrotizing granulomatous lymphadenitis was noted in some patients who had M simiae infection.[44]

Treatment

M simiae complex is resistant to many drugs normally used to treat tuberculosis. Antibiotics that have been reported to be effective include clarithromycin, ethambutol, ethionamide, fluoroquinolones, and amikacin.[45] The duration of treatment varies based on the treatment response and can be as long as 6 months to more than a year. Fine-needle aspiration is not recommended because of the risk for creating a chronically draining sinus tract.[30,31,45]

GROUP II: SCOTOCHROMOGENS
Mycobacterium Scrofulaceum

M scrofulaceum is a slow-growing scotochromogen that produces light yellow to orange pigment when exposed to both light and dark conditions. It is most prevalent in southeastern United States.[47] It has been isolated from raw milk and other dairy products, pooled oysters, soil, and water.[48] Cutaneous infections from M scrofulaceum are rare and usually are part of disseminated infection involving internal organs and the integumentary system. Immunocompromised patients, such as those who have AIDS, amyloidosis, hematologic malignancies, and those on immunosuppressive drugs, are at a higher risk.[48]

Clinical features

M scrofulaceum is acquired usually through inhalation or ingestion and most commonly presents as local lymphadenitis with fistulas in the submandibular or submaxillary region.[12] The most common site of NTM infection in children is the superficial lymph nodes of the head and neck.[49–52] M scrofulaceum was the most common cause of lymphadenitis in children until the 1970s when it was surpassed by MAI. M scrofulaceum is still responsible for 10% to 20% of unilateral cervical lymphadenitis.[28,53] The shift from M scrofulaceum to MAI could be because of the change in prevalence of M scrofulaceum in water.[53]

Lesions can also present as erythematous papules that slowly progress to ulcerated nodules.[48] Constitutional symptoms are usually absent.

Histopathology

Pathology is variable. It may demonstrate central necrosis and abscess formation surrounded by tuberculoid granuloma with considerable inflammatory cells composed of neutrophils, epithelioid histiocytes, and lymphocytes. Acid-fast bacilli are usually noted in the lymph node. Epidermal acanthosis and hyperkeratosis can be seen. PCR-ELISA can be beneficial in identifying the organism.[30,31,48]

Treatment

No clear guidelines for treating M scrofulaceum exist. Infections have been treated with quinolones, tetracyclines, and antituberculoid drugs, such as isoniazid, rifampin, and ethambutol.[23] Clarithromycin monotherapy was reported to be effective with no recurrences.[48] Surgical resection during the early stage of infection produced the most satisfactory healing in one report.[28]

Mycobacterium Szulgai

M szulgai is a scotochromogen that was first identified in 1972.[7,54] It is predominantly a pulmonary pathogen that affects patients regardless of preexisting pulmonary disease. The natural habitat is unknown but it can be found in snails and tropical fish. The organism has strong catalase positivity, positive nitrate and urease tests, and a delayed Tween hydrolysis reaction. It has a 2:1 male/female ratio. M szulgai is found in osteomyelitis, soft tissue infections, AIDS, and chronic lung disease.[55] M szulgai infection has also been reported in patients on anti–TNF-α therapy.[56]

Clinical features

M szulgai most commonly causes lung disease that may be mistaken for tuberculosis. It has been associated with COPD, smoking, and alcohol.[54] Cutaneous involvement has been along with other extrapulmonary infections, such as osteomyelitis, tenosynovitis, and lymphadenitis.[54]

Histopathology

Granulomas without caseation have been noted on pathology. As with other NTMs, culture of the biopsied tissue and PCR-ELISA can be beneficial in identifying the organism.[37]

Treatment

M szulgai infection has been effectively treated with triple drug therapy that included rifampicin, ethambutol, and clarithromycin.[56] Resistance has been reported in this organism to isoniazid, rifampin, and pyrazinamide, but it is sensitive to clarithromycin, doxycycline, ciprofloxacin, and amikacin.[57]

GROUP III: NONCHROMOGENS
Mycobacterium Avium-Intracellulare

M avium-intracellulare complex (MAC) consists of M avium, M intracellulare, and other unidentified species. Because it is not possible to differentiate between M avium and M intracellulare by normal biochemical means they are usually grouped together. The sensitization to M intracellulare was shown to be increasing by Khan and colleagues[58] from 1 in 9 people in 1971 to 1972 to 1 in 6 people in 1999 to 2000, which corresponded to the increased number of pulmonary NTM infections in the USA.

MAI is primarily a pulmonary pathogen and is the most commonly associated NTM species to cause human disease.[59] It has been isolated from chicken, swine, and feces from healthy individuals.[49] Inhalation of the organism causes pulmonary disease, whereas ingestion of contaminated water causes disseminated disease. Cutaneous manifestation can either be attributable to direct inoculation, direct contact, or part of disseminated disease.[12] It frequently involves the reticuloendothelial system, lung, bone, or skin.[59]

Clinical features

MAI causes pulmonary disease and is the most common cause of lymphadenitis in children accounting for around 80% to 90% of cases.[53] Lesions appear as painful or painless subcutaneous nodules in the cervical, submandibular, submaxillary, or preauricular region.[60] The nodules are usually unilateral and may ulcerate with discharge of a serosanguineous material. Systemic symptoms are usually absent. Deeper infections, such as panniculitis, synovitis, and fascitis, have also been reported.[12,60]

Histopathology

Granulomatous dermatitis with presence of macrophages containing large numbers of acid-fast bacilli in acute lesions is seen. Necrosis is usually absent.

Treatment

MAI infections must be treated aggressively. Clarithromycin, clofazimine, azithromycin, isoniazid, ethambutol, amikacin, rifampin, or rifabutin have been reported to be effective.[40] A multidrug regimen including clarithromycin 250 to 500 mg twice daily plus ethambutol 15 mg/kg/d plus rifampicin 600 mg daily has been suggested.[55] Streptomycin 1 g two to three times a week can be added for the first 2 months in severe cases. Azithromycin 250 to 500 mg three times a week, rifabutin 500 mg daily, and amikacin 1 g two to three times a week for first two months can also be used in place of clarithromycin, rifampicin, and streptomycin, respectively.[55]

Monotherapy with minocycline 100 mg twice a day for 1 yr was also successful. Pulmonary MAI should be treated until culture negative or 18 to 24 months.[55]

Mycobacterium Ulcerans

M ulcerans is a slow-growing nonchromogen that causes African Buruli ulcer and Bairnsdale ulcer. It is the most common NTM species causing disease worldwide.[60] It is not endemic to the Unite States and is found in tropical or warm temperate water bodies in Australia, Mexico, Africa, and Indonesia.[11,61] The organism grows at 32°C to 33°C and has a longer incubation period of 2 to 3 months. Children are affected more than adults. *M ulcerans* has a strong catalase reaction, negative nitrate reduction, negative niacin test, and a negative Tween hydrolysis.

Clinical features
M ulcerans enters the skin at sites of trauma, such as abrasions and cuts, and has a 2- to 3-month incubation period. The disease is more common in young patients and has a predilection for females. The lesions frequently present as a painless subcutaneous swelling, often on legs and forearms, that enlarges to form firm nodules.[61] Lesions may ulcerate and become necrotic. Mycolactone, a toxin produced by the organism, is believed to be responsible for the necrosis and suppression of the immune system.[60] Lesions spread rapidly and may involve deeper tissues.[12] Lesions often heal with scarring and contractures.

Histopathology
Granulomatous process with associated necrosis affecting predominantly subcutaneous fat is usually noted. Biopsy of the ulcerated area shows an extensive area of necrosis at the base with outline of normal tissue structure. Histology of deeper infection usually involves the subcutaneous fat but may involve the fascia, muscle, or bone. Leukocytoclastic vasculitis affecting small and medium-sized vessels is usually noted in the deeper dermis. Acid-fast bacilli are only noted during the acute stage of lesions and are found in the center of the lesion.[7] Culture of tissue biopsied and PCR-ELISA can be beneficial in identifying the organism.[30,31]

Treatment
Excision of the lesion at an early stage combined with grafting of the defect is the treatment of choice.[61] Pharmacotherapy can be combined with surgery for extensive disease. Local heat therapy is also of some benefit because the organism is heat sensitive.[61] Rifampin combined with amikacin (15 mg/kg IM twice daily) or streptomycin (15 mg/kg IM daily) with or without surgical therapy for 4 to 6 weeks has been suggested.[60]

Mycobacterium Haemophilum

M haemophilum is a nonchromogen that was first identified in 1978 by Sompolinsky in Israel in a woman who had Hodgkin disease who developed septic arthritis and skin lesions. It is more commonly seen in patients who have immunocompromised states, such as AIDS, hematologic malignancies, or chronic conditions that require prolonged immunosuppressive therapy. Cutaneous lesions are seen in more than 75% of patients who have *M haemophilum* infection.[28] *M haemophilum* grows at 30°C to 32°C and the growth medium must be supplemented with iron.[62]

Clinical features
M haemophilum affects adults and children after an inoculation period of around 2 to 3 weeks. Adults usually present with cutaneous lesions, bone involvement such as septic arthritis, or lung disease. In adults, multiple violaceous tender papules, plaques, or nodules are noted on the extremities, especially on the joints. Lesions may undergo abscess formation and ulceration.[12]

Children usually present with perihilar, cervical, or submandibular adenitis. Erythematous nodules with ulceration have been reported in children who have a history of renal transplant and are on immunosuppressive drugs, such as tacrolimus and prednisone.[63] Constitutional symptoms may be present.

Histopathology
The most common histologic pattern was a mixed suppurative and granulomatous reaction.[64,65] Acid-fast bacilli were found in 11 of 16 lesions. Four biopsies showed well-formed epithelioid granulomas. *M haemophilum* can present with nongranulomatous or pauci-granulomatous reactions without necrosis.[64] PCR-ELISA of the NTM hsp65 gene or sequencing of 16S rDNA can be beneficial in identifying the organism.[30,62,66–68]

Treatment
No clear guidelines exist for treating *M haemophilum* infections. The most active antimicrobial agents in vitro are amikacin, ciprofloxacin, clarithromycin, rifabutin, and rifampin.[62] Use of three-drug regimen containing a macrolide, a rifamycin, and a quinolone has been suggested. The duration and amount of therapy depends on the disease presentation and degree of immunosuppression.

Treatment for several months with at least two agents demonstrated to have low minimum inhibitory concentrations (MICs) for the organism has been shown to be effective.

GROUP IV: RAPID GROWERS
Mycobacterium Fortuitum

M fortuitum is a rapid grower that is widely distributed in the environment and found in soil, dust, water, milk, marine life, biofilm, and saliva of healthy humans.[12,40] Colonies are visible in 1 week or less. Outbreaks caused by rapid growers, such as *M fortuitum* and *M chelonei*, have been associated with jet injectors, hemodialysis, peritoneal dialysis, contaminated gentian violet skin-marking solution, catheters, prosthetic valves, surgical site infections, nail salons, full-face skin resurfacing with CO_2 laser, and contaminated injection solutions.[40,49,60,63,69] *M fortuitum* infections most commonly occur in immunocompetent individuals unlike *M chelonei* and *M abscessus*, which frequently cause disease in immunocompromised patients.[70] Winthrop and colleagues[72] reported an outbreak in 2002 in which more than 115 people contracted severe, lower extremity *M fortuitum* furunculosis from contaminated whirlpool footbaths used in a nail salon but only 32 were culture positive for *M fortuitum*.

Clinical features
Lesions develop after an inoculation period of 4 to 6 weeks. Soft tissue infections have been reported and are usually a result of surgery or penetrating trauma. Superficial manifestation is attributable to direct inoculation and is localized to the injury site. Lesions can vary from painful nodules, abscesses, ulcers, draining sinus tracts, or cellulitis. There should be clinical suspicion when patients present with nonhealing furuncles on the lower extremity and history should include possibility of recent pedicures.[70] Extracutaneous manifestations of *M fortuitum* and *M chelonei* can include postoperative vasculitis, endocarditis, osteomyelitis, mediastinitis, meningitis, keratitis, hepatitis, and bacteremia.[12,60,71]

Histopathology
Histopathology is variable and depends on the age of the lesion biopsied. Older lesions have a poor infiltrate, whereas acute lesions display suppurative granulomas without caseation, local tissue destruction, and a mixed infiltrate.[62] Suppurative folliculitis may be prevalent and acid-fast bacilli are usually absent in areas of chronic inflammation.[71]

Treatment
M fortuitum shows a high level of resistance to standard tuberculosis drugs. Clarithromycin and amikacin have been reported to be effective against some strains of *M fortuitum* in both immunocompromised and immunocompetent patients.[26] Winthrop and colleagues[72] suggested use of dual antibiotic therapy to minimize resistance. Many antibiotics, such as ciprofloxacin, doxycycline, minocycline, azithromycin, clarithromycin, and trimethoprim-sulfamethoxazole, have been reported to be effective; however, resistance to ciprofloxacin is emerging.[55,72] Surgical excision has been reported with satisfactory results to treat infections with rapid growers.[26]

A drug regimen consisting of doxycycline 100 mg daily, trimethoprim-sulfamethoxazole (800 mg-160 mg) twice daily, levofloxacin 500 to 750 mg daily, moxifloxacin 400 mg daily, or gatifloxacin 400 mg daily for 4 to 6 months has been suggested by Wagner and colleagues.[60]

Mycobacterium Chelonei

M chelonae is classified into three subspecies: *M chelonae chelonei*, *M chelonae abscessus*, and an unnamed subspecies known as *M chelonae*-like organism.[45] *M chelonei* is a rapid grower with colonies being visible as soon as 7 days. *M chelonae* was first isolated from the sea turtle, Chelonia corticata, after which it is named.

M chelonae is usually found in rivers, ponds, hot water springs, soil samples, and house dust. It can grow on Lowenstein-Jensen and MacConkey agar. It is known to contaminate injection solutions, along with *M fortuitum*, and cause soft tissue infections after cosmetic surgery, laparoscopic procedures, and other medical procedures.[62] *M chelonei* infections are also associated with prosthetic valves, catheters, and surgical sites.[60] Disseminated cutaneous infections have been noted to occur in patients who have rheumatoid arthritis and postrenal transplant.[28]

Clinical features
A common presentation is disseminated disease involving the distal aspect of a single extremity presenting as multiple erythematous nodules with draining fistulas. Lesions appear in a noncontiguous and nonlinear pattern. Localized disease following trauma or medical procedures, such as surgical site infection after chest surgery, is also common. Catheter-related infections involving central lines, drainage tubes, and prosthetic heart valves have also been reported.[55]

Cervical lymphadenitis has been reported. The nodes are usually described as of a rubbery consistency and focally matted with discharge through the overlying skin.[26]

Histopathology

Suppurative granulomas without caseation are usually noted on histology. The epidermis may show papillomatosis and hyperkeratosis. Inflammatory infiltrate, involving mostly neutrophils but also giant cells, and abscess formation involving the infundibulum were noted by Collina and colleagues.[30]

Treatment

M chelonei and M abscessus are identical genetically and phenotypically.[55] Standard tuberculosis drugs are ineffective because strains of M chelonei and M abscessus are usually resistant to them. Surgical débridement may be of some benefit but pharmacotherapy is usually needed. Minocycline monotherapy was reported to be successful against M chelonei and M abscessus.[62] Resistance to amikacin, cycloserine, doxycycline, vancomycin, and sulfisoxazole has been reported.[41] Surgical débridement combined with IV cefoxitin for 1 month and oral ciprofloxacin for 6 weeks has been reported to be effective with complete resolution.[41]

Mycobacterium Abscessus

M abscessus infection was first described in 1953 by Moore and Frerichs in a woman who had chronic osteoarthritis who developed a gluteal abscess. It is usually found in soil, water, and dust but it can also colonize body secretions and surfaces. Infections have been reported to occur after trauma, medical procedures such as augmentation mammoplasty, acupuncture, and injections.[73,74] Disseminated cutaneous infections have been noted to occur in patients who have immunosuppression secondary to other medical conditions, such as asthma, dermatomyositis, rheumatoid arthritis, and lupus erythematosus.[28] M abscessus is the most common NTM species causing infection in patients who have cystic fibrosis.[55]

Clinical features

Lesions appear as erythematous papules and pustules that later progress into ulcerated nodules. Lesions are more common on the lower extremities, followed by the upper extremities and trunk.[73] Ryu and colleagues[75] reviewed 40 cases of M abscessus infection acquired post-acupuncture. The most common site involved was the lower back with papules and nodules being the most common morphology.

Histopathology

Nodular or diffuse granulomatous pattern are the most common pathologic pattern.[76] The infiltrate in the specimen from immunocompromised patients tends to be deeper and involve the panniculus. Granulomatous suppurative inflammation without caseation was noted in 91.3% of patients reported by Tang and colleagues.[73] Rodriguez and colleagues[77] looked at biopsies from 71 patients who had M abscessus infections. A mixed lesion with abscesses surrounded by Langhans giant cells and epithelioid cells was seen in 80% of cases. Some 82% of biopsies revealed vacuolar spaces within the abscesses, surrounded by inflammatory cells. Acid-fast bacilli were noted in such spaces in 27% of these biopsies.[77]

Treatment

Clarithromycin monotherapy 500 mg twice daily has been reported to be effective with complete resolution in most patients (15 of 16 patients) in 12 months.[73]

SUMMARY

Atypical mycobacteria infections have been increasing over the past few decades and thus we have to be aware of their clinical presentation. Clinical features may vary from chronic localized skin infections to cervical lymphadenitis. The most common presentation in children is adenitis. Rapid growers, such as M fortuitum and M chelonei, may present as both cutaneous and lymph node infections, whereas M marinum only causes cutaneous disease. Biopsy should be done for histopathology diagnosis. Culture, special stains, and PCR can be helpful in identifying the organism. M marinum and M haemophilum grow at 28°C to 32°C, whereas most other NTM species grow at 35°C to 37°C. Also, the incubation period for M marinum is 2 to 8 weeks. It is important to let the laboratory know of any clinical suspicion so that the culture can be kept for an appropriate period of time to ensure that a proper identification is made. Steroid injections can exaggerate NTM infection and should be avoided.

REFERENCES

1. Jogi R, Tyring SK. Therapy of nontuberculous mycobacterial infections. Dermatol Ther 2004;17:491–8.
2. Ho MH, Ho CK, Chong LY. Atypical mycobacterial cutaneous infections in Hong Kong: 10-year retrospective study. Hong Kong Med J 2006;12(1):21–6.
3. Runyon EH. Anonymous mycobacteria in pulmonary disease. Med Clin North Am 1959;43:273–90.
4. Runyon EH. Pathogenic mycobacteria. Bibl Tuberc 1965;21:235–87.

5. Aronson JD. Spaontaneous tuberculosis in salt water fish. J Infect Dis 1926;39:315–20.

6. Norden A, Linell F. A new type of pathogenic mycobacterium. Nature 1951;168:826.

7. Groves R. Unusual cutaneous mycobacterial diseases. Clin Dermatol 1995;13:257–63.

8. Hautmann G, Lotti T. Diseases caused by Mycobacterium scrofulaceum. Clin Dermatol 1995;13:277–80.

9. Dalovisio JR, Pankey GA. Dermatologic manifestations of nontuberculous mycobacterial diseases. Infect Dis Clin North Am 1994;8(3):677–88.

10. Dodiuk-Gad R, Dyachenko P, Ziv M, et al. Nontuberculous mycobacterial infections of the skin: a retrospective study of 25 cases. J Am Acad Dermatol 2007;57:413–20.

11. Hautmann G, Lotti T. Atypical mycobacterial infections of the skin. Dermatol Clin 1994;12:657–68.

12. Weitzul S, Eichhorn PJ, Pandya A. Nontuberculous mycobacterial infections of the skin. Dermatol Clin 2000;18(2):359–77.

13. Brutus JP, Baeten Y, Kinnen CL, et al. Atypical mycobacterial infections of the hand: report of eight cases and literature review. Chir Main 2001;20:280–6.

14. Picó Moreno MR, Cruz A, Sánchez JL. Atypical mycobacterial infection. Bol Asoc Med P R 1989;81(6):206–8.

15. Harth M, Ralph ED, Faraawi R. Septic arthritis due to Mycobacterium marinum. J Rheumatol 1994;21(5):957–60.

16. Chopra N, Kirschenbaum AE, Widman D. Mycobacterium marinum tenosynovitis in a patient on etanercept therapy for rheumatoid arthritis. J Clin Rheumatol 2002;8(5):265–8.

17. Lam A, Toma W, Schlesinger N. Mycobacterium marinum arthritis mimicking rheumatoid arthritis. J Rheumatol 2006;33(4):817–9.

18. Rallis E, Koumantaki-Mathioudaki E, Frangoulis E, et al. Severe sporotrichoid fish tank granuloma following infliximab therapy. Am J Clin Dermatol 2007;8(6):385–8.

19. Salvana EM, Cooper GS, Salata RA. Mycobacterium other than tuberculosis (MOTT) infection: an emerging disease in infliximab-treated patients. J Infect 2007;55(6):484–7.

20. Kullavanijaya P. Atypical mycobacterial cutaneous infection. Clin Dermatol 1999;17:153–8.

21. Van Seymortier P, Verellen K, De Jonge I. Mycobacterium marinum causing tenosynovitis. "Fish tank finger". Acta Orthop Belg 2004;70(3):279–82.

22. Travis WD, Travis LB, Roberts GD, et al. The histopathologic spectrum in Mycobacterium marinum infection. Arch Pathol Lab Med 1985;109(12):1109–13.

23. Jackson JM. Emerging infections in dermatology. Semin Cutan Med Surg 2006;25(4):201–6.

24. Lotti T, Hautmann G. Atypical mycobacterial infections: a difficult and emerging group of infectious dermatoses. Int J Dermatol 1993;32(7):499–501.

25. Alinovi A, Vecchini F, Bassissi P. Sporothricoid mycobacterial infection. A case report. Acta Derm Venereol 1993;73(2):146–7.

26. Mahaisavariya P, Chaiprasert A, Khemngern S, et al. Nontuberculous mycobacterial skin infections: clinical and bacteriological studies. J Med Assoc Thai 2003;86(1):52–60.

27. Sagerman PM, Relman DA, Niroomand F, et al. Localization of Mycobacterium avium-intracellulare within a skin lesion of bacillary angiomatosis in a patient with AIDS. Diagn Mol Pathol 1992;1(3):212–6.

28. Bartralot R, García-Patos V, Sitjas D, et al. Clinical patterns of cutaneous nontuberculous mycobacterial infections. Br J Dermatol 2005;152(4):727–34.

29. Kullavanijaya P, Sirimachan S, Bhuddhavudhikrai P. Mycobacterium marinum cutaneous infections acquired from occupations and hobbies. Int J Dermatol 1993;32(7):504–7.

30. Collina G, Morandi L, Lanzoni A, et al. Atypical cutaneous mycobacteriosis diagnosed by polymerase chain reaction. Br J Dermatol 2002;147(4):781–4.

31. Hsiao PF, Tzen CY, Chen HC, et al. Polymerase chain reaction based detection of Mycobacterium tuberculosis in tissues showing granulomatous inflammation without demonstrable acid-fast bacilli. Int J Dermatol 2003;42(4):281–6.

32. Rajini M, Prasad SR, Reddy RR, et al. Postoperative infection of laparoscopic surgery wound due to Mycobacterium chelonae. Indian J Med Microbiol 2007;25(2):163–5.

33. Munayco CV, Grijalva CG, Culqui DR, et al. Outbreak of persistent cutaneous abscesses due to Mycobacterium chelonae after mesotherapy sessions. Lima, Peru. Rev Saude Publica 2008;42(1):146–9.

34. Morales P, Ros JA, Blanes M, et al. Successful recovery after disseminated infection due to mycobacterium abscessus in a lung transplant patient: subcutaneous nodule as first manifestation—a case report. Transplant Proc 2007;39(7):2413–5.

35. Morris-Jones R, Fletcher C, Morris-Jones S, et al. Mycobacterium abscessus: a cutaneous infection in a patient on renal replacement therapy. Clin Exp Dermatol 2001;26(5):415–8.

36. Hsu PY, Yang YH, Hsiao CH, et al. Mycobacterium kansasii infection presenting as cellulitis in a patient with systemic lupus erythematosus. J Formos Med Assoc 2002;101(8):581–4.

37. Li XJ, Wu QX, Zeng XS. Nontuberculous mycobacterial cutaneous infection confirmed by biochemical tests, polymerase chain reaction-restriction fragment length polymorphism analysis and sequencing of hsp65 gene. Br J Dermatol 2003;149(3):642–6.

38. Wolinsky E. Mycobacterial diseases other than tuberculosis. Clin Infect Dis 1992;15(1):1–10.

39. Wolinsky E. Mycobacterial lymphadenitis in children: a prospective study of 105 nontuberculous cases with long-term follow-up. Clin Infect Dis 1995;20(4): 954–63.

40. Katoch VM. Infections due to non-tuberculous mycobacteria (NTM). Indian J Med Res 2004;120(4): 290–304.

41. Plaus WJ, Hermann G. The surgical management of superficial infections caused by atypical mycobacteria. Surgery 1991;110(1):99–103.

42. Street ML, Umbert-Millet IJ, Roberts GD, et al. Nontuberculous mycobacterial infections of the skin. Report of fourteen cases and review of the literature. J Am Acad Dermatol 1991;24(2 Pt 1):208–15.

43. Cruz AT, Goytia VK, Starke JR. Mycobacterium simiae complex infection in an immunocompetent child. J Clin Microbiol 2007;45(8):2745–6.

44. Patel NC, Minifee PK, Dishop MK, et al. Mycobacterium simiae cervical lymphadenitis. Pediatr Infect Dis J 2007;26(4):362–3.

45. Conger NG, O'Connell RJ, Laurel VL, et al. Mycobacterium simae outbreak associated with a hospital water supply. Infect Control Hosp Epidemiol 2004; 25(12):1050–5.

46. Al-Abdely HM, Revankar SG, Graybill JR. Disseminated Mycobacterium simiae infection in patients with AIDS. J Infect 2000;41(2):143–7.

47. Sivasankari P, Khyriem A, Venkatesh K, et al. Atypical mycobacterial infection among HIV seronegative patients in Pondicherry. Indian J Chest Dis Allied Sci 2006;48:107–9.

48. Jang HS, Jo JH, Oh CK, et al. Successful treatment of localized cutaneous infection caused by Mycobacterium scrofulaceum with clarithromycin. Pediatr Dermatol 2005;22(5):476–9.

49. Starke JR. Nontuberculous mycobacterial infections in children. Adv Pediatr Infect Dis 1992;7:123–59.

50. Qunibi WY, al-Sibai MB, Taher S, et al. Mycobacterial infection after renal transplantation—report of 14 cases and review of the literature. Q J Med 1990; 77(282):1039–60.

51. Shah MK, Sebti A, Kiehn TE, et al. Mycobacterium haemophilum in immunocompromised patients. Clin Infect Dis 2001;33(3):330–7.

52. Saubolle MA, Kiehn TE, White MH, et al. Mycobacterium haemophilum: microbiology and expanding geographic spectra of disease in humans. Clin Microbiol Rev 1996;9:435–47.

53. Falkinham JO. The changing pattern of nontuberculous mycobacterial disease. Can J Infect Dis 2003; 14(5):281–6.

54. Meyer JJ, Gelman SS. Multifocal osteomyelitis due to Mycobacterium szulgai in a patient with chronic lymphocytic leukemia. J Infect 2008;56(2):151–4.

55. Petrini B. Non-tuberculous mycobacterial infections. Scand J Infect Dis 2006;38(4):246–55.

56. van Ingen J, Boeree M, Janssen M, et al. Pulmonary Mycobacterium szulgai infection and treatment in a patient receiving anti-tumor necrosis factor therapy. Nat Clin Pract Rheumatol 2007;3(7):414–9.

57. Kang-Birken SL, Prichard JG. Mycobacterium szulgai in a patient with advanced acquired immunodeficiency syndrome: an unusual pathogen with unusual multidrug resistance. Pharmacotherapy 2006;26(11):1646–9.

58. Khan K, Wang J, Marras TK. Nontuberculous mycobacterial sensitization in the United States: national trends over three decades. Am J Respir Crit Care Med 2007;176(3):306–13.

59. Friedman BF, Edwards D, Kirkpatrick CH. Mycobacterium avium-intracellulare: cutaneous presentations of disseminated disease. Am J Med 1988;85(2): 257–63.

60. Wagner D, Young LS. Nontuberculous mycobacterial infections: a clinical review. Infection 2004; 32(5):257–70.

61. Gart GS, Forstall GJ, Tomecki KJ. Mycobacterial skin disease: approaches to therapy. Semin Dermatol 1993;12(4):352–6.

62. Hutcheson AC, Lang PG. Atypical mycobacterial infections following cutaneous surgery. Dermatol Surg 2007;33(1):109–13.

63. Campbell LB, Maroon M, Pride H, et al. Mycobacterium haemophilum in an immunosuppressed child. Pediatr Dermatol 2006;23(5):481–3.

64. Busam KJ, Kiehn TE, Salob SP, et al. Histologic reactions to cutaneous infections by Mycobacterium haemophilum. Am J Surg Pathol 1999;23(11): 1379–85.

65. Kiehn TE, White M. Mycobacterium haemophilum: an emerging pathogen. Eur J Clin Microbiol Infect Dis 1994;13(11):925–31.

66. van Coppenraet LS, Smit VT, Templeton KE, et al. Application of real-time PCR to recognize atypical mycobacteria in archival skin biopsies: high prevalence of Mycobacterium haemophilum. Diagn Mol Pathol 2007;16(2):81–6.

67. Zumla A, Grange J. Infection and disease caused by environmental mycobacteria. Curr Opin Pulm Med 2002;8(3):166–72.

68. Gupta P, Katoch VM, Gupta UD, et al. A preliminary report on characterization and identification of non tuberculous mycobacteria (NTM) on the basis of biochemical tests and protein/isoenzyme electrophoretic patterns. Indian J Med Microbiol 2002; 20(3):137–40.

69. Rao J, Golden TA, Fitzpatrick RE. Atypical mycobacterial infection following blepharoplasty and full-face skin resurfacing with CO2 laser. Dermatol Surg 2002;28(8):768–71.

70. Redbord KP, Shearer DA, Gloster H, et al. Atypical Mycobacterium furunculosis occurring after pedicures. J Am Acad Dermatol 2006;54(3):520–4.

71. Sniezek PJ, Graham BS, Busch HB, et al. Rapidly growing mycobacterial infections after pedicures. Arch Dermatol 2003;139(5):629–34.

72. Winthrop KL, Albridge K, South D, et al. The clinical management and outcome of nail salon-acquired Mycobacterium fortuitum skin infection. Clin Infect Dis 2004;38(1):38–44.

73. Tang P, Walsh S, Murray C, et al. Outbreak of acupuncture-associated cutaneous Mycobacterium abscessus infections. J Cutan Med Surg 2006; 10(4):166–9.

74. Margileth AM. Management of nontuberculous (atypical) mycobacterial infections in children and adolescents. Pediatr Infect Dis 1985;4(2):119–21.

75. Ryu HJ, Kim WJ, Oh CH, et al. Iatrogenic Mycobacterium abscessus infection associated with acupuncture: clinical manifestations and its treatment. Int J Dermatol 2005;44(10):846–50.

76. Prinz BM, Michaelis S, Kettelhack N, et al. Subcutaneous infection with Mycobacterium abscessus in a renal transplant recipient. Dermatology 2004; 208(3):259–61.

77. Rodríguez G, Ortegón M, Camargo D, et al. Iatrogenic Mycobacterium abscessus infection: histopathology of 71 patients. Br J Dermatol 1997;137(2):214–8.

When Antibiotics are Unnecessary

J.V. Hirschmann, MD

KEYWORDS

- Antibiotics • Cutaneous abscess • Atopic eczema
- Prophylactic antibiotics • Cutaneous surgery

The use of antimicrobial agents when they are unwarranted exposes patients to several disadvantages: (1) adverse effects; (2) expense, which can be considerable, especially with the newer agents; and (3) risk for emergence of antimicrobial-resistant bacteria, both in patients and members of the wider community, to whom these organisms may be transmitted. Clinicians can obviate these potential problems by avoiding antibiotics in situations wherein careful studies have shown that they are unhelpful, which include several situations for which dermatologists commonly use them.

CUTANEOUS ABSCESSES

The bacteriology of cutaneous abscesses may have changed recently, but the general principles of therapy have not. In studies conducted in the 1970s to 1990s, investigators isolated *Staphylococcus aureus* from approximately 25% of cutaneous abscesses, usually in pure culture. It caused 40% or more of axillary and puerperal breast abscesses; approximately 20% to 40% of non-puerperal breast abscesses and abscesses on the trunk, extremities, buttocks, and inguinal areas; and fewer than 20% of abscesses on the head and neck and vulvovaginal, scrotal, and perineal areas.[1–8] Cutaneous abscesses not caused by *S aureus* were usually polymicrobial, with varying species of skin flora isolated from the pus, such as anaerobes and coagulase-negative staphylococci, often combined with bacteria colonizing nearby mucous membranes.

More recent studies suggest that *S aureus* causes approximately 65% to 75% of purulent skin and soft tissue infections, including cutaneous abscesses, with most isolates being methicillin-resistant *S aureus* (MRSA).[9–12] The increased rate of isolating MRSA compared with studies in the late 20th century may have arisen from investigating different patient populations or may indicate a genuine emergence of this organism as the preeminent contemporary cause of cutaneous abscesses. Support for the latter interpretation comes from the fact that MRSA seems to be a more virulent organism than methicillin-susceptible *S aureus* (MSSA), and its presence on the skin may lead to more infections than when MSSA is present.

Treatment of cutaneous abscesses remains incision and drainage. In four randomized controlled trials, the addition of an antibiotic to this procedure did not lead to a clinically significant improvement in outcome, although three studies preceded the emergence of MRSA. In an investigation involving 64 patients who had boils and abscesses, dicloxacillin given for 5 days did not significantly hasten healing compared with a control group that did not receive an antibiotic.[13] A second trial involving 219 abscesses also found no difference in healing time between patients initially receiving lincomycin and then clindamycin for 4 days compared with those not undergoing antimicrobial therapy.[14]

In the third study, which included 50 participants, wound healing was equivalent at the end of therapy whether patients received cephradine or a placebo for 7 days.[15] The fourth study, a double-blind trial in 166 patients, found no benefit with cephalexin 500 mg four times daily for 7 days compared with placebo.[12] In this investigation, most of the isolates were MRSA and therefore inherently resistant to cephalexin. Nevertheless, the cure rate was 90% in the placebo group, similar to what occurred in the earlier cephradine study (96%), conducted when MRSA was not present in the community.

Medical Service (111), Puget Sound VA Medical Center, 1660 South Columbian Way, Seattle, WA 98108, USA
E-mail address: pepsi@u.washington.edu

Dermatol Clin 27 (2009) 75–83
doi:10.1016/j.det.2008.07.003
0733-8635/08/$ – see front matter. Published by Elsevier Inc.

Furthermore, several retrospective studies have shown that, among patients who underwent incision and drainage for MRSA cutaneous abscesses, those who underwent antimicrobial therapy to which the organism was not susceptible had excellent outcomes equivalent to those who received antibiotics active against MRSA.[14,16,17] Although a 2005 survey indicated that 87% of health care providers prescribe antibiotics after incising and draining cutaneous abscesses,[18] overall evidence indicates that this antimicrobial therapy is unnecessary.

Inflamed Epidermal Cysts

Clinicians commonly mistake inflamed epidermal (often erroneously called *sebaceous*) cysts for abscesses, and even when they are recognized accurately, they are frequently assumed to be infected. This conclusion is understandable, because they are typically painful, fluctuant, warm, and red masses that, when incised and drained, often yield pus and their usual cheesy, malodorous contents. The presence of inflammation and pus does not necessarily indicate infection, however, and cultures of 25 inflamed and 25 uninflamed cysts showed that the number and types of bacteria were similar in both groups.[19] Anaerobes and coagulase-negative staphylococci were common, but *S aureus* grew from only 3 (6%) cysts. This study indicates that inflammation of epidermal cysts is not from infection but probably from rupture of the cysts or leakage of contents through their wall into the adjacent tissue, provoking an intense inflammatory response. Similar to cutaneous abscesses, appropriate therapy is incision and drainage without antibiotics.

VENOUS ULCERS

Cultures of leg ulcers that form from venous insufficiency yield a wide variety of bacteria, even in the absence of obvious features of infection, such as fever or substantial surrounding cellulitis.[20–24] The isolates are potentially pathogenic; approximately 30% grow *S aureus*, 15% *Streptococcus* spp, 25% enteric gram-negative bacilli, 20% *Pseudomonas* spp, and 5% other gram-negative bacilli. A critical issue is whether the presence of these organisms impairs resolution of the ulcers and, therefore, if antimicrobial therapy might hasten healing.

One trial determined whether a 10-day course of systemic antibiotics selected specifically for the organisms isolated had any effect on the course of the ulcers in 47 patients.[21] Local care, provided to all participants, consisted of antiseptic solution, corticosteroid cream, and compressive bandages.

Among the 23 patients receiving antibiotics, ulcer healing at day 20 was not greater than for the 24 control patients. In another trial of more protracted systemic antimicrobial therapy, 12 subjects received oral ciprofloxacin, 9 trimethoprim, and 10 placebo for 12 weeks.[22] Neither antibacterial agent improved the rate of healing, but both markedly encouraged colonization with drug-resistant organisms. In the ciprofloxacin recipients, 94% of the bacteria isolated at the end of the study were resistant compared with 12% in the trimethoprim group and 4% in the placebo group. For subjects receiving trimethoprim, 65% of the bacteria isolated at 12 weeks were resistant, as were 63% of the isolates among those receiving ciprofloxacin, compared with only 8% of those from the placebo group. These studies indicate that systemic antimicrobial therapy for uninfected venous ulcers does not accelerate healing but does encourage colonization with drug-resistant organisms.

Diabetic Foot Ulcers

As with venous ulcers, diabetic foot ulcers have a rich microbiology even without clinical evidence of infection, which is typically defined by the presence of surrounding soft-tissue inflammation, including erythema, heat, induration, and swelling. Cultures of clinically stable, uninfected ulcers yield an average of approximately five bacterial species (approximately three facultative and two anaerobic). The most frequent isolates include enteric gram-negative bacilli, *P aeruginosa*, *S aureus*, various streptococci, coagulase-negative staphylococci, and anaerobes.[25]

As with venous ulcers, a critical clinical issue is whether these bacteria impair wound healing. In a study of 44 patients experienced forefoot neuropathic diabetic ulcers, ranging from superficial to deep (reaching joint or tendon), administering amoxicillin-clavulanate for 20 days did not have any effect on ulcer healing compared with those receiving placebo.[26] The number of patients with complete closure of the ulcer at 20 days was 10 of 12 in the placebo group compared with 6 of 12 of those receiving antibiotics, and the median daily reduction in ulcer diameter was 0.41 mm in those receiving placebo compared with 0.27 mm in the antibiotic group. All patients received equivalent local wound care. Therefore, similar to venous ulcers, antimicrobial therapy of superficial diabetic foot ulcers does not accelerate wound healing.

ATOPIC ECZEMA

S aureus resides in the nose and on the skin in a large percentage of patients who have atopic eczema. It is present in the nares in approximately 60% of cases, on the affected skin in approximately 85%, and on the uninvolved skin in approximately 60%.[27–32] Whether these staphylococci are just colonizing organisms or pathogens is debated. Some investigators have asserted that the concentration of the bacteria is critical, and when *S aureus* exceeds a density of 10^6 per cm^2 on the involved skin, it exacerbates the disease.[29] Numerous studies have shown that topical (neomycin,[29] gentamicin,[33] and mupirocin[32]) and systemic antimicrobials (erythromycin,[29] flucloxacillin,[27] and cephalexin[34]) can decrease the number of *S aureus*, but the effects of these interventions on the eczema itself have been variable, providing either no improvement[27] or mild benefit.[29,32–34] The reduction or eradication of *S aureus*, however, was transient; the organism recolonized the skin within a few weeks after discontinuing the antimicrobial therapy.[27,32,34] A serious consequence with flucloxacillin, at least, was the emergence of drug-resistant bacteria during or after treatment.[27]

Reduction of the density of *S aureus* also occurs with topical corticosteroids, which have no inherent antimicrobial activity but, unlike topical and systemic antimicrobials, consistently produce substantial clinical improvement.[35,36] This outcome does not arise from the properties of the steroid's vehicle. In a double-blind trial, desonide had substantial bacteriologic and clinical benefits, but the excipient was ineffectual.[36] Furthermore, the reduction in the number of staphylococci and the improvement of the eczema increased with the potency of the corticosteroid. Clobetasol, a very powerful steroid, was better than clobetasone and alclometasone, which are moderately potent agents.[35] These investigations indicate that the concentration of staphylococci increases with the intensity of the inflammation and that reducing inflammation alone decreases the number of colonizing organisms.

Several trials have examined whether the combination of topical antimicrobial and corticosteroid produces better results than corticosteroids alone. In a study of impetiginized eczema, topical gentamicin was less effective than betamethasone valerate, and the combination was no better than the steroid by itself.[33] In a group of infected or potentially infected eczema, betamethasone valerate alone was equivalent to its combination with fusidic acid, an antimicrobial with good activity against staphylococci.[37] In a small study, fluocinolone and neomycin were better than the steroid alone, and hydrocortisone plus polymyxin B, neomycin, and gramicidin was superior to the topical antibiotics alone.[38] In several trials of infected

eczema, mupirocin was more effective than its vehicle, but the combination of it and topical corticosteroids was not superior to the steroids alone.[39] In one trial of patients who had no overt secondary infection, however, mupirocin plus topical corticosteroids was better than steroids alone.[32]

Two trials investigated the use of systemic antibiotics in atopic eczema. When patients received topical corticosteroids, flucloxacillin produced no additional benefit.[27] When patients received no topical corticosteroids, those treated with cephalexin experienced better results than controls, because the antibiotic resulted in a mild clinical improvement.[34]

A reasonable conclusion from these various investigations is that topical or systemic antistaphylococcal agents provide, at best, minor clinical benefit in patients who receive no topical corticosteroids, but proper therapy of atopic eczema must include medications that reduce inflammation, such as corticosteroids. When patients appropriately receive topical corticosteroids, adding topical or systemic antimicrobial therapy is, at most, minimally helpful, and may encourage the emergence of drug-resistant organisms and increase medical care costs. Recognizing the presence of infection in atopic eczema may seem perplexing when erythema, weeping, and crusting occur, but these studies indicate that such features alone do not justify antimicrobial therapy. Antibiotics in atopic eczema are clearly warranted only in the presence of unambiguous signs of infection (eg, fever, pustules, cellulitis, lymphangitis).[40]

Antimicrobial Prophylaxis to Reduce Postoperative Wound Infections in Dermatologic Surgery

The bacteriology of infections after dermatologic surgery remains ill-defined, but most pathogens apparently arise from a patient's own resident cutaneous or mucosal flora. When the organisms enter the wound, they may induce local inflammation or, rarely, invade the bloodstream, causing metastatic foci of infection or the findings of symptomatic bacteremia, such as fever and hypotension. The organisms causing these infections are typically present on the skin adjacent to the surgical site, sometimes accompanied by microbes from nearby mucous membranes. The most important resident cutaneous flora include coryneform bacteria, anaerobes, and coagulase-negative staphylococci, such as *S epidermidis*. Although each of these bacteria alone is weakly pathogenic, they may cause infection when present together in a wound. In addition, *S aureus* is present in the nose or, less commonly, the throat in approximately 20% to 40% of normal adults, and colonizes intertriginous areas, such as the perineum, in up to 20%.[41] From these home bases, S aureus can travel to adjacent or distant skin areas and cause infection alone or as a component of a mixed flora when cutaneous injuries occur, including surgical procedures. The major elements of postoperative infections in dermatologic surgery, therefore, are S aureus and the normal cutaneous bacteria.

Determining whether antimicrobials are justified in trying to prevent postoperative wound infections in dermatologic surgery depends on understanding the classification of operations and their anticipated rates of infection. The most prevalent scheme identifies four types of procedures: clean, clean-contaminated, contaminated, and dirty (or infected).[42] Clean surgery, which constitutes approximately 75% of all operations, involves no inflammation or entry into the respiratory, genitourinary, or gastrointestinal tracts. The expected postoperative wound infection rate is less than 5% and is usually approximately 1% to 2%. Clean-contaminated surgery, which constitutes about 15% of procedures, enters the respiratory, genitourinary, or gastrointestinal tract, but no significant spillage occurs. The wound infection rate is approximately 10%, but can be much greater with certain procedures, especially colorectal surgery. Contaminated operations involve acute nonpurulent inflammation, gross spillage from the gastrointestinal tract, a major break in sterile technique, fresh trauma, or entry into infected biliary or urinary tracts. The expected infection rate is about 20%. Dirty or infected surgery includes traumatic wounds with retained, devitalized tissue, foreign bodies, fecal contamination, or already infected tissues. Postoperative wound infections occur in approximately 30% to 40% of cases.

The major principles of antimicrobial prophylaxis in surgery are:[42]

(1) Virtually all wound infections arise from contamination of the surgical site during the operation, with responsible organisms usually from adjacent cutaneous or mucosal surfaces.
(2) The antibacterial agent used must be active against most of the usual pathogens; its purpose is not to annihilate the entire contaminating flora but to reduce the microbial population to a low level at which clinical infection is unlikely to occur.
(3) The antimicrobial must be present in the tissue when the wound contamination occurs or shortly thereafter; regimens that initiate prophylaxis later are ineffectual.
(4) Because contamination usually ends when the wound is closed, postoperative antimicrobials are unnecessary; a single preoperative or intraoperative dose of the agent almost always suffices.

To justify surgical antimicrobial prophylaxis, the procedure must have one of two characteristics:

(1) Its infection rate is so high that antimicrobial prophylaxis results in less antibiotic use than if no prophylaxis occurred. An example is colorectal surgery, in which a single dose of a preoperative antibiotic reduces the postoperative infection rate from approximately 40% to 5%.[43–45] Because the infections that develop usually require several days of antimicrobial therapy, the overall antimicrobial use for treating patients who did not receive prophylaxis exceeds the amount used for prevention.
(2) The incidence of infection is low, but its effects are so catastrophic that an overall economic benefit occurs from antimicrobial prophylaxis. An example is prosthetic joint insertion. In one study, antimicrobial prophylaxis only slightly decreased the postoperative hip infection rate, from approximately 3% to 1%.[46] The cost of preventing a single prosthetic infection, however, exceeds the cost of the prophylactic antimicrobials for hundreds of patients, because these infections typically require removing the prosthesis, several weeks of antimicrobial therapy, protracted hospitalization, and reinsertion of another artificial joint.

Dermatologic procedures satisfy neither of these criteria. The overall wound infection rate is low. A summary of four studies including approximately 6000 dermatologic operations shows an incidence of about 1.3%.[47–50] Among Mohs' micrographic procedures, the rate is approximately 2.5%. Moreover, most of these infections are mild and easily managed, commonly with wound care alone and no antibiotics. Systemic antimicrobial prophylaxis can further reduce this low infection rate,[51] but the benefits do not justify the costs, including expense of the medications, risks for adverse drug effects, and potential for encouraging antibiotic resistance among the infecting organisms.

Some types of dermatologic procedures have more frequent infections, or the infections have more serious consequences than others. In these circumstances, intraincisional injection of a very low dose of antibiotic is an attractive alternative to systemic agents. Using 0.5 mg/mL of nafcillin injected approximately 15 minutes preoperatively along with 1% buffered lidocaine and epinephrine 1:100,000 into the anticipated surgical incision site led to a wound infection rate of 0.2% compared with 2.5% in those receiving lidocaine and epinephrine, a statistically significant difference.[49] This randomized, double-blind trial involved 908 wounds from Mohs' surgery, the second part of any staged repair, and the excision of benign cutanecus neoplasms.

These authors conducted a similar trial in 1172 wounds, all involving Mohs' surgery with reconstruction, using clindamycin 40 μg/mL with the same concentration of lidocaine and epinephrine as in the previous study.[50] The wound infection rate in patients treated with clindamycin was 0.8% compared with 2.7% with those in the placebo group, also a statistically significant difference. Compared to oral, intravenous, or intramuscular administration, the use of these miniscule amounts of antibiotic delivered directly to the wound has the advantages of convenience, decreased cost, and little systemic effect, with, therefore, a low likelihood of adverse drug reactions, medication interactions, and encouragement of antimicrobial resistance among patients' flora.

A common method of antimicrobial prophylaxis is applying a topical antimicrobial on the suture site. Because most wound infections result from contamination before wound closure, however, this approach is ineffective. An unpublished study of neomycin compared with its ointment base showed no reduction in infections.[39]

A randomized, double-blind trial comparing white petrolatum compared with bacitracin ointment applied daily for 7 to 10 days to 1207 wounds showed an infection rate of 1.5% in the former group compared with 0.9% in the latter, a statistically insignificant difference.[52] In the white petrolatum group, almost all infections were from S aureus, whereas all were caused by gram-negative bacilli in the bacitracin group. Contact dermatitis occurred in 0.9% of the bacitracin group, compared with none in the white petrolatum group. Adding the contact dermatitis rate to the wound infection rate, the incidence of wound complications was higher in the bacitracin group: 1.8% versus 1.5%. The bacitracin ointment was fourfold more expensive than the white petrolatum, and even considering the costs of systemic antimicrobials to treat the wound infections, the medication costs for the patients were still 3.5 times higher, because the infecting bacteria required more expensive agents for therapy. Moreover, the wound healing time was equal in both groups. Therefore, bacitracin ointment is no better than white petrolatum in dermatologic surgery and is more expensive, can cause contact dermatitis, promotes wound infections with resistant bacteria, and does not accelerate healing.

One study examined 778 patients who had uninfected skin undergoing punch biopsy, elliptic incision, incisional biopsy, full- and partial-thickness skin grafts, and random pattern skin flaps.[53] Patients randomly received no ointment, sterile paraffin (Lacri-Lube), or mupirocin on the wound before having it covered with a moist occlusive dressing. No differences were seen in the rate of infection, scar, dehiscence, or hemorrhage. The frequency of skin necrosis, however, was statistically significantly higher in the patients treated with mupirocin. This study shows that when moist occlusive dressings are used, no ointment is necessary for the wound after dermatologic surgery, and the use of mupirocin is actually harmful.

Antibiotics to Prevent Endocarditis Following Cutaneous Surgery

The 2007 American Heart Association (AHA) guidelines do not recommend antimicrobial administration to prevent endocarditis in any patients undergoing dermatologic surgery unless it involves already infected skin, soft tissue, or musculoskeletal structures.[54] Moreover, the guidelines restrict prophylaxis to patients who have four types of cardiac conditions: (1) a history of endocarditis, (2) prosthetic valves or prosthetic material used for cardiac valve repair, (3) previous cardiac transplantation with subsequent development of cardiac valvulopathy, and (4) certain kinds of congenital heart diseases, such as patients who have unrepaired cyanotic heart disease, including those who have palliative shunts and conduits; completely repaired congenital heart disease with prosthetic material or device inserted within the past 6 months; or repaired congenital heart disease with residual defects at or adjacent to the site of a prosthetic patch or device.

The recommended prophylactic oral regimens relevant to dermatologic surgery, to be taken as a single dose 30 to 60 minutes before the procedure, include either cephalexin, 2 g, or clindamycin, 600 mg (adult doses). For patients unable to take oral medications, the parenteral regimens include a single dose, administered 30 to 60 minutes before the procedure, of cefazolin or ceftriaxone, 1 g, intramuscularly or intravenously; clindamycin, 600 mg, intramuscularly or intravenously; or vancomycin, 1 g, intravenously.

The 2007 AMA recommendations primarily address dental procedures and represent a major change from the previous guidelines in markedly restricting potential candidates for antimicrobial prophylaxis to the four categories listed above. This change was made for several reasons: very few cases of endocarditis result from medical or dental procedures, the efficacy of antimicrobial prophylaxis in preventing these cases was never proved, there are potential adverse effects, and the chances of developing endocarditis vary according to the cardiac condition, allowing prophylaxis to be confined to those at highest risk.

For dermatologists, the risk of causing endocarditis from a procedure is extremely small for several reasons. First, the incidence of bacteremia, which is the necessary precursor for endocarditis to develop, is low in dermatologic surgery. In five studies including 279 patients,[55–59] 5 (1.8%) had positive blood cultures: one with S aureus, two with coagulase-negative staphylococci, and two with Propionibacterium acnes. This rate is nearly identical to that recorded in a study of 240 healthy people, in whom 2.1% of blood cultures were positive, mostly with coagulase-negative staphylococci.[60] These isolates in normal people almost certainly represent contamination of the cultures by skin organisms at venipuncture, as do the coagulase-negative staphylococci and the P acnes (a cutaneous organism of very low virulence), grown from the blood of patients undergoing dermatologic surgery in the studies cited above.

Therefore, among the 279 patients, a reasonably common pathogen for endocarditis—the isolate of S aureus—was present in the blood cultures of only 1 (0.3%). This rate of bacteremia is extraordinarily low to justify giving preoperative antibiotics for routine dermatologic surgery, even to patients at the highest risk for cardiac lesions, especially compared with the 95% rate of positive cultures for potential pathogens in patients undergoing certain dental procedures and the common occurrence of transient bacteremia in daily activities.[61] For example, the rates of bacteremia with organisms that commonly cause endocarditis are approximately 40% for tooth brushing or dental irrigation, 20% for chewing bubble gum, 20% for dental flossing, and 15% for chewing hard candy.[61]

Certain dermatologic procedures, however, may have higher rates of bacteremia than others. Debriding of bed sores in eight patients caused positive blood cultures in five (62%), with some specimens yielding more than one species, but nearly all isolates were organisms highly unlikely to produce endocarditis.[62] They were anaerobes in five cases, gram-negative bacilli in four, and group B streptococcus in one—the only organism that causes endocarditis with any frequency.

Abscess manipulation is another situation that might cause a high rate of bacteremia. A study from the preantibiotic era involved gently massaging furuncles caused by S aureus for 10 minutes.[63] In 5 of 13 patients (38%), transient bacteremia occurred. The relevance of this finding for surgery is unclear, but it suggests that pressure on an abscess, which probably occurs frequently during daily activities, might cause numerous episodes of bacteremia and be more likely to produce endocarditis than the single event of incision and drainage.

The actual incidence of transient bacteremia from surgical treatment of skin abscesses is unclear; the two published reports provide strikingly different results. In one study, 6 of 10 patients had positive blood cultures, yielding a total of 19 isolates, but 14 were bacteria that rarely cause endocarditis (12 anaerobes and 2 gram-negative bacilli).[64] The remaining 4 isolates were gram-positive cocci, but none was S aureus (P. Scheckman, personal communication, 2003).

Another study of 50 afebrile patients who had cutaneous abscesses in various locations detected no instances of bacteremia after incision and drainage.[65] Together these studies suggest that bacteremia with organisms commonly causing endocarditis rarely occurs from surgical treatment of skin abscesses. Nevertheless, the AMA guidelines suggest antimicrobial prophylaxis in this situation for patients who have the high-risk cardiac conditions mentioned earlier.

Although perhaps prudent, this recommendation is based on almost no data. The causative association of any prior procedures and the subsequent development of endocarditis is only conjecture, but few reports of endocarditis have implicated dermatologic procedures. As of 1993, only four existed, and none has been published since, at least in the English language literature.[66] The putative procedures in these cases were incisional skin biopsy, cryotherapy, punch biopsy, and melanoma excision. None was from incision and drainage of a cutaneous abscess. Furthermore, one case-control study found that staphylococcal endocarditis was not related to surgeries.[67]

Antibiotics to Prevent Infections of Noncardiac Prostheses

Giving antimicrobial prophylaxis for routine dermatologic procedures in patients who have noncardiac prostheses is unwarranted. Infection of prosthetic joints and vascular grafts through hematogenous spread from a distant site is uncommon. When it does occur, nearly all cases arise from an established focus of infection rather than from transient bacteremia related to a medical or dental procedure. For example, in a prospective study of 1000 patients who underwent joint replacement and a subsequent follow-up for 6 years, only 3 had hematogenous infections, all related to concurrent suppuration elsewhere.[68] In the 224 who underwent a dental or operative procedure without antimicrobial prophylaxis, no infections developed.

A compilation of 180 reported cases of hematogenous infections of joint replacements as of 1996 indicated that only 11 were from a dermatologic procedure, and at least 5 of these involved an already infected site.[69] In some of the remaining 7 cases, the authors did not state whether infection was present, and the relationship between the procedure and the subsequent infection may have been coincidental.

Experimentally, joint and vascular prostheses become infected only with high-level bacteremia, far greater than occurs after medical and dental procedures, and both types of devices become increasingly difficult to infect as time elapses after implantation.[70–72] This information indicates that antimicrobial prophylaxis for dermatologic surgery involving uninfected tissue is unnecessary in patients who have noncardiac prostheses. However, when surgery involves incision of infected tissue, the infection should be treated appropriately before the procedure.

SUMMARY

Current evidence indicates that antibiotics are usually unnecessary in patients who have cutaneous abscesses, even those caused by MRSA. Instead, appropriate therapy involves incision and drainage alone. That procedure, again without concurrent antimicrobial therapy, is also indicated for inflamed epidermal cysts. Unless substantial surrounding soft-tissue inflammation is present, topical or systemic antimicrobial therapy is not indicated for venous or diabetic ulcers. Topical or systemic antimicrobial therapy is also not indicated for atopic dermatitis, despite the common presence of S aureus on inflamed skin, unless there is clear evidence of infection, such as pustules, cellulitis, or lymphangitis.

Prophylactic antibiotics are rarely necessary for patients who have cardiac disease undergoing dermatologic surgery, and clinicians should follow the 2007 AMA guidelines. Furthermore, no evidence supports the use of preventive antimicrobials in patients who have vascular grafts or orthopedic prostheses undergoing routine dermatologic surgery. Topical antibiotics are no better than white petrolatum for use on sutured incisions after cutaneous surgery. When moist occlusive dressings are used, no ointment is necessary.

REFERENCES

1. Meislin HW, Lerner SA, Graves MH, et al. Cutaneous abscesses. Anaerobic and aerobic bacteriology and outpatient management. Ann Intern Med 1977;87:145–9.
2. Brook I, Frazier EH. Aerobic and anaerobic bacteriology of wounds and cutaneous abscesses. Arch Surg 1990;125:1445–51.
3. Whitehead SM, Leach RD, Eykyn SJ, et al. The aetiology of scrotal sepsis. Br J Surg 1982;69:729–30.
4. Leach RD, Eykyn SJ, Phillips I, et al. Anaerobic axillary abscess. Br Med J 1979;2:5–7.
5. Leach RD, Eykyn SJ, Phillips I, et al. Anaerobic subareolar abscess. Lancet 1979;1:35–7.
6. Ghoneim ATM, McGoldrick J, Blick PWH, et al. Aerobic and anaerobic bacteriology of subcutaneous abscesses. Br J Surg 1981;68:498–500.
7. Edmiston CE, Walker AP, Krepel CJ, et al. The nonpuerperal breast infection: aerobic and anaerobic microbial recovery from acute and chronic disease. J Infect Dis 1990;162:695–9.
8. Whitehead SM, Eykyn SJ, Phillips I. Anaerobic paronychia. Br J Surg 1981;68:420–2.
9. Fridkin SK, Hageman JC, Morrison M, et al. Methicillin-resistant Staphylococcus aureus disease in three communities. N Engl J Med 2005;352:1436–44.
10. Moran GJ, Krishnadasan A, Gorwitz RJ, et al. Methicillin-resistant S aureus infections among patients in the emergency department. N Engl J Med 2006;355:666–74.
11. Frazee BW, Lynn J, Charlebois ED, et al. High prevalence of methicillin-resistant Staphylococcus aureus in emergency department skin and soft tissue infections. Ann Emerg Med 2005;45:311–20.
12. Rajendran PM, Young D, Maurer T, et al. Randomized, double-blind, placebo-controlled trial of cephalexin for treatment of uncomplicated skin abscesses in a population at risk for community-acquired methicillin-resistant Staphylococcus aureus infection. Antimicrobial Agents Chemother 2007;51:4044–8.
13. Rutherford WH, Calderwood JW, Hart D, et al. Antibiotics in surgical treatment of septic lesions. Lancet 1970;1:1077–80.
14. Macfie J, Harvey J. The treatment of acute superficial abscesses: a prospective clinical trial. Br J Surg 1977;64:264–6.
15. Llera JL, Levy RC. Treatment of cutaneous abscess: a double-blind clinical study. Ann Emerg Med 1985;14:15–9.
16. Lee MC, Rios AM, Aten MF, et al. Management and outcome of children with skin and soft tissue abscesses caused by community-acquired methicillin-resistant Staphylococcus aureus. Pediatr Infect Dis J 2004;23:123–7.
17. Paydar KZ, Hansen SL, Charlebois ED, et al. Inappropriate antibiotic use in soft tissue infections. Arch Surg 2006;141:850–6.
18. Rajendran PM, Young D, Maurer T, et al. Antibiotic use in the treatment of soft tissue abscesses: a

survey of current practice. Surg Infect (Larchmt) 2007;8:237–8.

19. Diven DG, Dozier SE, Meyer DJ, et al. Bacteriology of inflamed and uninflamed epidermal inclusion cysts. Arch Dermatol 1998;134:49–51.

20. Erickson G, Eklund AE, Kallinger LO. The clinical significance of bacterial growth in venous leg ulcers. Scand J Infect Dis 1984;16:175–80.

21. Alinovi A, Bassissi P, Pini M. Systemic administration of antibiotics in the management of venous ulcers: a randomized clinical trial. J Am Acad Dermatol 1986;15:186–91.

22. Hansson C, Hoborn J, Moller A, et al. The microbial flora in venous leg ulcers without clinical signs of infection. Repeated culture using a validated standardized microbiological technique. Acta Derm Venereol 1995;75:24–30.

23. Gilchrist B, Reed C. The bacteriology of chronic venous ulcers treated with occlusive hydrocolloid dressings. Br J Dermatol 1989;121:337–44.

24. Pardes JB, Carson PA, Eaglstein WH, et al. Mupirocin treatment of exudative venous ulcers. J Am Acad Dermatol 1993;29:497–8.

25. Louie TJ, Bartlett JG, Tally FP, et al. Aerobic and anaerobic bacteria in diabetic foot ulcers. Ann Intern Med 1976;85:461–3.

26. Chantelau E, Tanudjaja T, Altenhofer F, et al. Antibiotic treatment for uncomplicated neuropathic forefoot ulcers in diabetes: a controlled trial. Diabet Med 1996;13:156–9.

27. Ewing CI, Ashcroft C, Gibbs ACC, et al. Flucloxacillin in the treatment of atopic dermatitis. Br J Dermatol 1998;138:1022–9.

28. Aly R, Maibach HI, Shinefield HR. Microbial flora of atopic dermatitis. Arch Dermatol 1977;113:780–2.

29. Leyden JJ, Marples RR, Kligman AM. Staphylococcus aureus in the lesions of atopic dermatitis. Br J Dermatol 1974;90:525–30.

30. Goodyear HM, Watson PJ, Egan SA, et al. Skin microflora of atopic eczema in first time hospital attenders. Clin Exp Dermatol 1993;18:300–4.

31. Masenga J, Garbe C, Wagner J, et al. Staphylococcus aureus in atopic dermatitis and in nonatopic dermatitis. Int J Dermatol 1990;29:579–82.

32. Lever R, Hadley K, Downey D, et al. Staphylococcal colonization in atopic dermatitis and the effect of topical mupirocin therapy. Br J Dermatol 1988;119:189–98.

33. Wachs GN, Maibach HI. Co-operative double-blind trial of an antibiotic/corticoid combination in impetiginized atopic dermatitis. Br J Dermatol 1976;95:323–8.

34. Breuer K, Haussler S, Kapp A, et al. Staphylococcus aureus: colonizing features and influence of an antibacterial treatment in adults with atopic dermatitis. Br J Dermatol 2002;147:55–61.

35. Nilsson EJ, Henning CG, Magnusson J. Topical corticosteroids and Staphylococcus aureus in atopic dermatitis. J Am Acad Dermatol 1992;27:29–34.

36. Stalder JF, Fleury M, Sourisse M, et al. Local steroid therapy and bacterial skin flora in atopic dermatitis. Br J Dermatol 1994;131:536–40.

37. Hjorth N, Schmidt H, Thomsen K. Fusidic acid plus betamethasone in infected or potentially infected eczema. Pharmatherapeutica 1985;4:126–31.

38. Leyden JJ, Kligman AM. The case for steroid-antibiotic combination. Br J Dermatol 1977;96:179–87.

39. Hirschmann JV. Topical antibiotics in dermatology. Arch Dermatol 1988;124:1691–700.

40. Hanifin JM, Rogge JL. Staphylococcal infections in patients with atopic dermatitis. Arch Dermatol 1977;113:1383–6.

41. Roth RR, James WD. Microbiology of the skin: Resident flora, ecology, infection. J Am Acad Dermatol 1989;20:367–90.

42. Hirschmann JV. Antimicrobial prophylaxis in dermatology. Semin Cutan Med Surg 2000;19:2–9.

43. Eykyn SJ, Jackson BT, Lockhart-Mummery HE, et al. Prophylactic preoperative intravenous metronidazole in elective colorectal surgery. Lancet 1979;2:761–4.

44. Feathers RS, Lewis AAM, Sagor GR, et al. Prophylactic systemic antibiotics in colorectal surgery. Lancet 1977;2:4–8.

45. Portnoy J, Kagan E, Gordon PH, et al. Prophylactic antibiotics in elective colorectal surgery. Dis Colon Rectum 1983;26:310–3.

46. Hill C, Flamant R, Mazas F, et al. Prophylactic cefazolin versus placebo in total hip replacement. Report of a multicentre double-blind randomised trial. Lancet 1981;1:795–7.

47. Futoryan T, Grande D. Postoperative wound infection rates in dermatologic surgery. Dermatol Surg 1995;21:509–14.

48. Whitaker DC, Grande DJ, Johnson SS. Wound infection rate in dermatologic surgery. J Dermatol Surg Oncol 1988;14:525–8.

49. Griego RD, Zitelli JA. Intra-incisional prophylactic antibiotics for dermatologic surgery. Arch Dermatol 1998;134:688–92.

50. Huether MJ, Griego RD, Brodland DG, et al. Clindamycin for intraincisional antibiotic prophylaxis in dermatologic surgery. Arch Dermatol 2002;138:1145–8.

51. Bencini PL, Galimberti M, Signorini M, et al. Antibiotic prophylaxis of wound infections in skin surgery. Arch Dermatol 1991;127:1357–60.

52. Smack DP, Harrington AC, Dunn C, et al. Infection and allergy incidence in ambulatory surgery patients using white petrolatum vs bacitracin ointment. A randomized controlled trial. JAMA 1996;276:972–7.

53. Dixon AJ, Dixon MP, Dixon JB. Randomized clinical trial of the effect of applying ointment to surgical

wounds before occlusive dressing. Br J Surg 2006; 93:937–43.

54. Wilson W, Taubert KA, Gewitz M, et al. Prevention of infective endocarditis. Guidelines from the American Heart Association. Circulation 2007;116:1736–54.

55. Sabetta JB, Zitelli JA. The incidence of bacteremia during skin surgery. Arch Dermatol 1987;123:213–5.

56. Halpern AC, Leyden JJ, Dzubow LM, et al. The incidence of bacteremia in skin surgery of the head and neck. J Am Acad Dermatol 1988;19:112–6.

57. Zack L, Remlinger K, Thompson K, et al. The incidence of bacteremia after skin surgery. J Infect Dis 1989;159:148–50.

58. Maurice PDL, Parker S, Azadian BS, et al. Minor skin surgery. Are prophylactic antibiotics ever needed for curettage? Acta Derm Venereol 1991;71:267–8.

59. Carmichael AJ, Flanagan PG, Holt PGA, et al. The occurrence of bacteraemia with skin surgery. Br J Dermatol 1996;134:120–2.

60. Wilson WR, Van Scoy RE, Washington JA. Incidence of bacteremia in adults without infection. J Clin Microbiol 1975;2:94–5.

61. Hirschmann JV. Antimicrobial prophylaxis in dermatologic surgery. Cutis 2007;79(Suppl):43–51.

62. Glenchur H, Bhupendrakumar SP, Pathmarajah C. Transient bacteremia associated with debridement of decubitus ulcers. Mil Med 1981;146:432–3.

63. Richards JH. Bacteremia following irritation of foci of infection. JAMA 1932;99:1496–7.

64. Fine BC, Sheckman PR, Bartlett JC. Incision and drainage of soft-tissue abscesses and bacteremia. Ann Intern Med 1985;103:645.

65. Bobrow BJ, Pollack CV, Gamble S, et al. Incision and drainage of cutaneous abscesses is not associated with bacteremia in afebrile adults. Ann Emerg Med 1997;29:404–8.

66. Spelman DW, Weinmann A, Spicer WJ. Endocarditis following skin procedures. J Infect 1993;26:185–9.

67. Lacassin F, Hoen B, Leport C, et al. Procedures associated with infective endocarditis in adults. A case control study. Eur Heart J 1995;16:1968–74.

68. Ainscow DAP, Denham RA. The risk of haematogenous infection in total joint replacements. J Bone Joint Surg [Br] 1984;66:580–2.

69. Deacon JM, Pagliaro AJ, Zelicof SB, et al. Prophylactic use of antibiotics for procedures after total joint replacement. J Bone Joint Surg 1996;78A:1755–70.

70. Malone JM, Moore WS, Campagna G, et al. Bacteremic infectability of vascular grafts: The influence of pseudointimal integrity and duration of graft function. Surgery 1975;78:211–6.

71. Southwood RT, Rice JL, McDonald PJ, et al. Infection in experimental hip arthroplasties. J Bone Joint Surg 1985;67B:229–31.

72. Blomberg G. Hematogenous infection of total joint replacement An experimental study in the rabbit. Acta Orthop Scand 1981;52(Suppl 187):1–64.

Use of Antibiotics for Noninfectious Dermatologic Disorders

Neal Bhatia, MD

KEYWORDS

• Antibiotics • Inflammation • Dermatology

One fascinating element of medical dermatology is the diversity of available therapeutic agents, and dermatologists are well versed in applying the mechanism of action of a drug to modify a disease process. Oral antibiotics are the ideal example of pharmacologic agents that are effective against inflammatory processes and have obvious roles in infectious diseases.

Aside from the well-known uses of antibiotics in common conditions such as acne, rosacea, and perioral dermatitis, many applications of various antibiotics could be made part of the dermatologists' routine. Although the current reality of prescribing antibiotics faces challenges of insurance formularies, patient inquiries, and concern for resistance and superinfections (eg, methicillin-resistant *Staphylococcus aureus*), the potential benefits in certain disease states far outweigh the negative answers to questions about their initiation.[1]

ANTI-INFLAMMATORY ACTIVITY

Inflammation patterns that affect epidermal turnover, infiltrative processes, and destruction of dermal constituents can all be influenced by the effects of agents on leukocytes and dendritic cells that start the patterns. In addition, long-term countering of inflammation to avoid sequelae requires consistent suppression of the cell lines involved. Most antibiotics used in dermatology for noninfectious conditions affect the 30S ribosome (tetracyclines), 50S ribosome (macrolides), or important steps in DNA replication (fluoroquinolones, rifampin, and sulfones). Most other families of commonly used antibiotics, such as penicillins, cephalosporins, and carbapenems, act on specific components of bacterial cell wall synthesis and therefore have limited applications for inflammatory dermatoses.[1]

TETRACYCLINES

Aside from the common uses in acne and rosacea, which can mainly be attributed to activity against *Propionibacterium acnes*, the tetracycline family of antibiotics has a diverse usefulness in dermatology. Mechanisms of action include inhibition of granulomas and proteases, effects on chemotaxis, activities against protein kinase C, and angiogenesis. As a result, they have many potential uses as anti-inflammatory agents, especially minocycline, which has shown efficacy in multiple disorders.[2]

CONFLUENT AND RETICULATED PAPILLOMATOSIS

Confluent and reticulated papillomatosis (CRP) of Gougerot and Carteaud is an uncommon disorder of unknown cause. Endocrine disturbances show increased turnover of cells in response to therapies that regulate cell development and prevent skin cell growth. Clearance with antifungal treatment has also been suggested because of presence of *Malassezia* spp organisms in some CRP cases. In addition, some CRP cases respond to antibacterial treatment. Recently an actinomycete called *Dietzia* was reportedly isolated from a patient who had confluent and reticulated papillomatosis.[3] Dietzia strain xL is a newly described Actinomycete isolated from confluent and reticulated papillomatosis.

A case report described the effectiveness of oral minocycline on nine patients who had CRP treated

University of Wisconsin Medical School, Madison, WI, USA
E-mail address: ndbhatia@juno.com

Dermatol Clin 27 (2009) 85–89
doi:10.1016/j.det.2008.07.007
0733-8635/08/$ – see front matter © 2009 Elsevier Inc. All rights reserved.

with oral minocycline, 50 mg twice daily for 6 weeks. The average follow-up period was 11 months. All patients except two experienced a 90% to 100% response to therapy. Recurrences were noted in three patients, who all responded to re-treatment with minocycline.[4]

Another case review discusses six cases of CRP alleviated with various antibiotics. The patient described in one case was a 16-year-old girl successfully treated with minocycline, 100 mg daily for 8 weeks. Cases 2 and 3 describe an 18-year-old woman and a 17-year-old male adolescent who experienced improvement on oral fusidic acid, 1000 mg daily for 4 weeks. Another case involved a 14-year-old girl who received oral clarithromycin, 500 mg daily for 5 weeks, and experienced moderate changes. The last two patients were a 22-year-old woman whose disease was reduced with oral erythromycin, 1000 mg daily for 6 weeks, and a 24-year-old man who received oral azithromycin, 500 mg daily three times per week for 3 weeks. These improvements with antibiotic treatment further support the possibility that CRP is triggered by a bacterial infection, suggesting that antibiotics are the preferred treatment for CRP.[5]

SILICONE GRANULOMA OF THE FACE TREATED WITH MINOCYCLINE

One case report discussed treatment of a 43-year-old woman who had a severely disfiguring facial silicone granuloma and underwent successful treatment with minocycline. Siliconoma represents a granulomatous foreign body reaction to silicone, used for soft tissue augmentation. Treatment of siliconomas and similar granulomas involving the face are examples of how the diverse mechanisms of action of minocycline can be applied.[6]

PIGMENTED POSTACNE OSTEOMA CUTIS IN A PATIENT TREATED WITH MINOCYCLINE

Postacne osteoma cutis is a rare complication of acne vulgaris. If it occurs during a course of tetracycline or minocycline therapy, pigmented osteomas can occur as a result of tetracycline or minocycline bone complexes. The authors report a case of pigmented postacne osteoma cutis that developed after extensive acne surgery and a 2- to 3-month course of minocycline. Previously reported cases have been treated surgically, but the authors' patient responded to 0.05% tretinoin cream, with transepidermal elimination of some osteomas.[7]

MELKERSSON-ROSENTHAL SYNDROME IN CHILDHOOD: COMBINATION STEROID AND MINOCYCLINE

The Melkersson-Rosenthal syndrome involves the triad of recurrent lip or face swelling, fissured tongue, and intermittent facial palsy. One case report described two children who had Melkersson-Rosenthal syndrome in whom combination treatment with prednisone and minocycline proved effective and well tolerated in reducing the symptom complex.[8]

TREATMENT OF RECURRENT AURICLE PSEUDOCYST WITH INTRALESIONAL INJECTION OF MINOCYCLINE: A REPORT OF TWO CASES

Pseudocyst of the auricle (PCA) is characterized by asymptomatic and fluctuant swelling of the external ear and frequent relapses despite various therapeutic approaches. Two patients who had recurrent PCA were successfully treated with two or three intralesional injections of 1 mg/mL of minocycline hydrochloride (minocycline) given at 2-week intervals. Intralesional injection of minocycline may be a new therapeutic choice for conservative management of PCA, especially in recurrent cases.[9]

TETRACYCLINES HELP CHRONIC CUTANEOUS SARCOIDOSIS

A small study by Bachelez and colleagues[10] evaluated the safety and efficacy of minocycline in treating sarcoidosis. Twelve patients who had cutaneous sarcoidosis were treated with minocycline, 200 mg/d, for a median duration of 12 months. Complete clearing of lesions was noted in 8 of 12 patients who had cutaneous sarcoidosis, with a median follow-up of 26 months. A slight hyperpigmentation occurred in two patients at the site of previous lesions, which completely disappeared after minocycline was discontinued. A relapse of skin symptoms occurred after minocycline withdrawal in three patients, who then received doxycycline, 200 mg/d, allowing complete remission of lesions. Clinical response, defined as regression of at least 50% of lesions, was seen in 10 patients.

MINOCYCLINE DECREASES SEVERITY OF CETUXIMAB RASH

Cetuximab is an epidermal growth factor (EGFR) inhibitor that is used to treat metastatic colorectal cancer. However, cetuximab produces an acne-like rash in more than 80% of patients treated. Although an effective treatment for rashes linked to EGFR inhibitors is not available, severe cetuximab-related eruptions have been controlled through interrupting treatment or reducing the dose.

One study involved 48 patients who were about to start cetuximab who received oral minocycline 100 mg daily or placebo for 8 weeks in addition to topical tazarotene to prevent cetuximab-associated acneiform rash. Patients were randomized to oral minocycline or oral placebo, along with open-label tazarotene applied to one side of the face, beginning on the same day as cetuximab initiation. Lesion counts were significantly lower in patients treated with minocycline than in those treated with placebo. Patients treated with minocycline were also less likely than placebo patients to report moderate to severe itch and rash.[11]

MINOCYCLINE IN EARLY DIFFUSE SCLERODERMA

In an uncontrolled trial involving 11 patients who had early but severe diffuse scleroderma, oral minocycline was well tolerated and seemed to improve skin manifestations in four of six patients who completed a year of treatment. Expanded studies are warranted. Treatment with minocycline was initiated at 50 mg twice daily, and the dose was increased to 100 mg twice daily after 1 month. This protocol was used to avoid the dizziness or headache occasionally encountered by patients who have rheumatoid arthritis when starting on minocycline.[12]

Other common antibiotics have been used in conditions with variable results, but their applications and usefulness are to provide possible options for patients when other therapies either have failed or are not indicated. In addition, antimicrobial effects may apply when a bacterial nature of the disease has not been excluded.

PITYRIASIS ROSEA

Isolated reports of improvement of pityriasis rosea in two patients receiving erythromycin led to a 2-year double-blind, placebo-controlled study involving 90 patients. These subjects were alternatively assigned to treatment group or placebo group. Patients in the treatment group received erythromycin in divided doses for 14 days. The response was categorized as complete response, partial response, or no response. All patients were followed up for 6 weeks. Upper respiratory tract infection before the appearance of skin lesions was reported in 68.8% of all patients. Complete response was observed in 33 patients (73.33%) in the treatment group and none in the placebo group ($P<.0001$).[13]

Clarithromycin was also discussed as effective therapy in patients who have pityriasis rosea given its potential for improvement with fewer gastrointestinal effects. A study performed in Greece involved 64 patients who had pityriasis rosea randomized three-to-one to a 12-day course of clarithromycin 250 mg twice daily in adults and 15 mg/kg per day in children or no therapy. Patients treated with placebo showed a slow resolution within 6 to 8 weeks, as opposed to 45 of 48 patients treated with clarithromycin that showed regression of their skin lesions by the end of week 1 and were completely clear of lesions and symptom-free after 4 weeks.[14]

BALANITIS XEROTICA OBLITERANS

Three patients who had balanitis xerotica obliterans were reported to have significant improvement after long-term antibiotics. Two patients treated with oral and intramuscular penicillin noticed softening of the skin and disappearance of pruritus, tenderness, and inflammatory changes within 3 weeks, whereas a third patient improved after a regimen of 500 mg/d of dirithromycin. Discontinuing the antibiotic for 1 month resulted in relapse, with improvement on resumption.[15,16]

ORAL LICHEN PLANUS

In a series of patients who had desquamative gingivitis, six who had oral lichen planus were treated with doxycycline monohydrate at 100 mg daily for 3 weeks. One patient improved dramatically, three improved slightly, and two were either unchanged or worse after the therapy. The benefits of this drug are most likely from its anti-inflammatory action and not its antibacterial activity. Although early investigators suggested a bacterial origin for lichen planus, electron microscopy and cultures failed to reveal bacteria.[17] Another case report provided a similar efficacy with tetracycline.[18]

BULLOUS DERMATOSES

Use of tetracyclines in adjunctive roles for bullous dermatoses, such as bullous pemphigoid and pemphigus, has been well documented and remains a mainstay of chronic therapy. In combination with nicotinamide, tetracycline helps reduce toxicity of steroids and other immunosuppressive drugs. Historically, the bullae and lesions of bullous pemphigoid primarily contain neutrophils, eosinophils, and histamine, which is consistent with the fact that tetracycline and nicotinamide inhibit neutrophil and eosinophil chemotaxis, and nicotinamide has antihistamine effects at the receptor and inhibits histamine release. These mechanisms are likely involved in the therapeutic effect seen with these drugs.[19] Although other derivatives in the tetracycline family have not supplanted use of the original compound, minocycline and doxycycline have been substituted, although risks for photosensitivity, vestibular side effects, and hyperpigmentation, among the other potential long-term adverse outcomes associated with these drugs, limit their efficacy.

One of the more controlled studies comparing the combination of tetracycline and nicotinamide with prednisone alone involved 20 patients randomized by a ratio of 14:6 into each group. The patients treated with the combination of nicotinamide 500 mg three times daily and tetracycline 500 mg four times daily were compared against those receiving variable oral steroid doses between 40 and 80 mg every day. In the first 8 weeks of the trial, five patients in the nicotinamide/tetracycline group had complete responses, five patients experienced partial responses, one had no change, and one experienced disease progression. Two patients were lost to follow-up. In the prednisone-treated group, one patient experienced a complete response and five had partial responses. Eight patients were available for long-term follow-up; two of the three available patients treated with prednisone and only one of the five available patients treated with nicotinamide/tetracycline experienced flares of the disease while medications were being tapered.[19] Several patients developed gastrointestinal toxicity and nephrotoxicity, which resulted in a change of therapy to minocycline.

Concerns about using minocycline instead of tetracycline include potential for pigmentation, vestibular side effects, and gastrointestinal toxicity. A review involving the use of minocycline 50 or 100 mg daily for various bullous disorders, including pemphigus vulgaris, pemphigus foliaceous, and bullous pemphigoid, showed that hyperpigmentation was a limiting step in its long-term use. Seven of nine patients treated with minocycline, 50 mg daily (one patient) or 100 mg twice daily (eight patients), developed hyperpigmentation, although five of these patients improved with minocycline therapy. Average treatment duration was 8.2 months (range, 1–25 months). Oral candidiasis was also observed in two patients.[20]

Several case reports have been published on antibiotic use as adjunctive therapy for linear IgA dermatosis (chronic bullous of childhood). One report reviewed the course of seven patients who had linear IgA dermatosis of childhood treated with flucloxacillin. In four patients, the agent induced complete remission within 3 to 4 months with no relapses. In the other three cases, it successfully controlled the disease but with prompt relapse on discontinuation of treatment.[21] Another case report on the use of erythromycin in linear IgA disease in adults and children suggests similar success in reducing the need for other aggressive immunosuppressive therapies.[22] Finally, dicloxicillin has also been reported to be a possible therapeutic option in chronic bullous of childhood.[23]

SUMMARY

As more derivatives of existing antibiotics are created, such as incyclinide in the tetracycline family, longer-acting minocycline capsules, or other compounds similar to erythromycin that are gastrointestinal-protective, the application of antibiotics as anti-inflammatory agents or adjunctive therapies to steroids may become more common in dermatology regimens. These compounds probably have more potential roles in dermatology aside from their traditional uses in treating of acne and rosacea, but this will require matching the mechanism of the drug to the disease process.

REFERENCES

1. Wolverton S. Comprehensive dermatologic drug therapy. Philadelphia: WB Saunders; 2001. p. 28–54.
2. Webster G. Anti-Inflammatory activity of tetracyclines. Dermatol Clin 2007;25(2):133–5.
3. Natarajan S, Milne D, Jones AL, et al. Dietzia strain X: a newly described actinomycete isolated from confluent and reticulated papillomatosis. Br J Dermatol 2005;153:825–7.
4. Montemarano AD, Hengge M, Sau P, et al. Confluent and reticulated papillomatosis: response to minocycline. J Am Acad Dermatol 1996;34(2 Pt 1):253–6.
5. Jang H, et al. Six cases of confluent and reticulated papillomatosis alleviated by various antibiotics. J Am Acad Dermatol 2001;44:652–5.
6. Arin MJ, Bäte J, Krieg T, et al. Silicone granuloma of the face treated with minocycline. J Am Acad Dermatol 2005;52(2):S53–6.
7. Moritz DL, Elewski B. Pigmented postacne osteoma cutis in a patient treated with minocycline: report and review of the literature. J Am Acad Dermatol 1991;24(5 Pt 2):851–3.
8. Stein S, Mancini A. Melkersson-Rosenthal syndrome in childhood: successful management with combination steroid and minocycline therapy. J Am Acad Dermatol 1999;41:746–8.

9. Oyama N, Satoh M, Iwatsuki K, et al. Treatment of recurrent auricle pseudocyst with intralesional injection of minocycline: a report of two cases. J Am Acad Dermatol 2001;45:554–6.

10. Bachelez H, et al. Tetracyclines help chronic cutaneous sarcoidosis. Arch Dermatol 2001;137(1):69–73.

11. Gould P. Minocycline in early diffuse scleroderma. Lancet Oncol 2008;9(1):17.

12. Le CH, Morales A, Trentham D. Lancet 1998; 352(9142):1755–6.

13. Sharma P, et al. Erythromycin in pityriasis rosea: a double-blind, placebo-controlled clinical trial. J Am Acad Dermatol 2000;42:241–4.

14. Karpouzis A. Clarithromycin offers relief in pityriasis rosea. Internal Medicine News 2004;vol 37(6):73.

15. Shelley WB, et al. Long-term antibiotic therapy for balanitis xerotica obliterans. J Am Acad Dermatol 1999;40:69–72.

16. Ronbeck BA, Lind PO, Thrane PS. Desquamative gingivitis: preliminary observations with tetracycline treatment. Oral Surg Oral Med Oral Pathol 1990; 69:694–7.

17. Whitten JB. Intraoral lichen planus simplex: an ultrastructure study. J Periodontol 1970;41: 261–4.

18. Chan J. Tetracyclines in the treatment of lichen planus. J Am Acad Dermatol 2007;vol. 56(Issue 2): AB62.

19. Fivenson DP, et al. Nicotinamide and tetracycline therapy of bullous pemphigoid. Arch Dermatol 1994;130:753–8.

20. Ozog DM, Gogstetter DS, Scott G, et al. Minocycline-induced hyperpigmentation in patients with pemphigus and pemphigoid. Arch Dermatol 2000; 136:1133–8.

21. Abdulmajeed A, et al. Treatment of linear IgA bullous dermatosis of childhood with flucloxacillin. J Am Acad Dermatol 54(4):652–6.

22. Cooper SM, Powell J, Wojnarowska F. Linear IgA disease: successful treatment with erythromycin. Clin Exp Dermatol 2002;27(8):677–9.

23. Siegfried EC, Sirawan S. Chronic bullous disease of childhood: successful treatment with dicloxacillin. J Am Acad Dermatol 1998;39(5 Pt 1):797–800.

Oral Antibiotic Drug Interactions of Clinical Significance to Dermatologists

James Q. Del Rosso, DO, FAOCD*

KEYWORDS

- Oral antibiotics • Drug interactions
- Enzyme induction • Enzyme inhibition

Oral antibiotics are commonly prescribed in dermatology practice for various cutaneous infections and for noninflammatory disorders, such as acne vulgaris and rosacea.[1] Dermatologists prescribe approximately 8 to 9 million oral antibiotic prescriptions annually based on data collected over a 5-year time period (2001–2005), with tetracycline agents accounting for approximately 60% of total prescriptions.[2] The efficacy of antibiotic therapy depends on adequate systemic absorption of the administered agent. As a result, decreased antibiotic absorption from the gastrointestinal (GI) tract because of concomitant ingestion of another drug or ingestant may decrease antibiotic efficacy. Additionally, metabolic drug–drug interactions may affect potential toxicity if there is inhibited metabolism of one concurrently administered drug by another. This article reviews selected drug interactions associated with the use of oral antibiotics that may be of clinical significance to the dermatologist.

DRUG INTERACTIONS MECHANISMS

Drug interactions can occur through several potential mechanisms related to altered absorption, metabolism, distribution, or excretion.[3] The mechanisms most often associated with drug interactions of potential clinical significance are (1) altered GI absorption of antibiotic and (2) inhibition or induction of drug metabolism.[3–5] Specific examples related to these mechanisms are discussed below.

DRUG INTERACTION DYNAMICS

Drug interactions occur commonly; however, in many cases their effects represent a pharmacologic nuance and do not result in clinically significant outcomes.[3–5] It is only when a drug interaction produces a pharmacodynamic effect that correlates with decreased drug efficacy or systemic toxicity that the interaction is of clinical consequence.

Drug interactions that produce recognizable toxicity are more likely to be detected by the cognizant clinician. An example of such a drug interaction would be development of rhabdomyolysis secondary to impaired hepatic metabolism of atorvastatin by erythromycin.[6] Drug interactions that result in reduced efficacy are more likely to remain unrecognized. An example is reduced GI absorption of ciprofloxacin secondary to concurrent use of an antacid or mineral supplement containing aluminum, magnesium, calcium, or iron resulting in antibiotic treatment failure.[7] These metal ions chelate ciprofloxacin and several other quinolone antibiotics in the GI tract, thus impairing their absorption and subsequent access to the systemic circulation. In this scenario, the clinician is likely to believe that the ciprofloxacin was simply not effective, not considering that it was the drug interaction that caused the lack of efficacy.

DRUG INTERACTIONS AFFECTING GASTROINTESTINAL ABSORPTION

The most common type of oral antibiotic drug interaction related to GI tract drug absorption

Valley Hospital Medical Center, 620 Shadow Lane, Las Vegas, NV 89106, USA
* 880 Seven Hills Drive, Suite 260, Henderson, NV 89052.
E-mail address: jqdelrosso@yahoo.com

Dermatol Clin 27 (2009) 91–94
doi:10.1016/j.det.2008.07.011

that is of potential clinical significance is chelation of the antibiotic by concurrently ingested metal ions.[3–5] Such metal ions may include calcium, aluminum, magnesium, and iron, which may be found in vitamin-mineral supplements, or, in some cases, antacids (ie, calcium carbonate, aluminum hydroxide, magnesium sulfate). Attempting to optimally separate the ingestion times between the antibiotic and metal ions may reduce the extent of interaction; however, this tends to be variable depending on the specific ion and antibiotic. A reasonable guideline to follow is to administer the oral antibiotic at least 1 to 2 hours before, and not within 4 hours after, the ingested metal ions, assuming it is not clinically feasible to discontinue the use of the product containing the metal ions. Additionally, food products know to contain high concentrations of calcium, such as milk and yogurt, are best avoided in a similar fashion.

Tetracyclines

Coadministration of tetracycline with several metal ions, such as calcium, magnesium, aluminum, zinc, or bismuth, has been reported to markedly reduce the GI absorption of tetracycline.[8,9] Reduced efficacy of tetracycline may ensue.

Ingestion of tetracycline with milk or yogurt is best avoided. Although co-ingestion with a meal does not seem to significantly reduce the GI absorption of doxycycline or minocycline, concurrent use of iron may reduce GI absorption of doxycycline or minocycline.[8,10] Bismuth subsalicyclate may markedly reduce the GI absorption of doxycycline.[9] The clinical significance of the extent of chelation of doxycycline or minocycline by iron is not entirely clear; however, avoidance if clinically feasible is a reasonable recommendation.

Quinolones

The GI absorption of several quinolone antibiotics, such as ciprofloxacin, may be reduced by concurrent administration of calcium, aluminum, or magnesium.[7,11] Concurrent ingestion of calcium with ciprofloxacin within less than 15 minutes has been shown to reduce ciprofloxacin absorption by 40%.[11] Ingestion of ciprofloxacin within 4 hours after an aluminum- or magnesium-containing antacid has been reported to reduce ciprofloxacin absorption by approximately three fourths.[11] The extent of reduction of individual quinolone antibiotics secondary to concomitant use of products containing specific metal ions is variable, making it complicated for the clinician to realistically remember all the interaction details. A practical guideline to follow in clinical practice is to administer the quinolone antibiotic at least 1 to 2 hours before, and not within

4 hours after, the ingested metal ions, assuming it is not clinically feasible to discontinue the use of the product containing the metal ions.[11]

DRUG INTERACTIONS AFFECTING HEPATIC METABOLISM

Drug interactions that occur because of modifications of hepatic metabolism relate to either enzyme inhibition or enzyme induction.[3–5,12] Enzyme inhibition occurs when the metabolism of one drug is inhibited by another drug that is being administered concurrently. The enzymes that are most commonly affected are components of the cytochrome P450 (CYP 450) metabolic enzyme system and include enzyme families, such as CYP3A4, CYP2D6, CYP 2C, and CYP 1A2.[3–5,12] The most common CYP 450 enzyme involved in inhibition drug interactions is CYP3A4, which represents a primary route of metabolism for approximately 50% of drugs available in the marketplace.[3–5,12] Enzyme induction occurs when the metabolism of one drug is increased by another drug that is being administered concurrently. CYP 3A4 is the most common enzyme system involved in induction drug interactions.[3–5,12]

What is the Potential Clinical Consequence of an Enzyme Inhibition Drug Interaction?

When the metabolism of a drug is inhibited, its serum level, and subsequently its bioavailability, is increased because of drug accumulation over time.[3–5] Toxicity may ensue if the extent of drug accumulation produces pharmacodynamic activity that creates clinically apparent side effects. An example of a clinically significant enzyme inhibition interaction is decreased hepatic metabolism of atorvastatin, simvastatin, or lovastatin by ketoconazole or itraconazole because of inhibition of CYP3A4, resulting in the development of rhabdomyolysis attributable to systemic accumulation of the statin agent.[13,14]

What is the Clinical Consequence of an Enzyme Induction Drug Interaction?

When the metabolism of a drug is increased, its serum level, and subsequently its bioavailability, is reduced because of enhanced metabolic conversion of active drug into its inactive metabolites. Treatment failure may ensue if increased drug metabolism produces a diminution of the level of active drug below the threshold needed to produce adequate therapeutic effect at the target tissue site. An example of a clinically significant enzyme induction interaction is oral contraceptive failure secondary to increased metabolism of estrogen caused by coadministration of rifampin.[15,16]

Macrolides

Erythromycin, and to a lesser extent clarithromycin, may produce clinically significant drug interactions through inhibition of CYP 3A4.[3–6,12] As a result, these agents should be avoided in patients receiving certain HMG-CoA reductase inhibitors (cholesterol-lowering agents) that are metabolized by CYP 3A4, such as atorvastatin, simvastatin, and lovastatin.[6] The potentially severe clinical consequence of decreased metabolism of these cholesterol-lowering agents is rhabdomyolysis.

Multiple cases of carbamazepine toxicity have been reported secondary to coadministration of erythromycin.[17–19] Erythromycin, and to a lesser extent clarithromycin, inhibit the hepatic metabolism of carbamazepine by the CYP 3A4 enzyme system. Carbamazepine toxicity secondary to concurrent use of erythromycin is associated with dizziness, vertigo, somnolence, and ataxia, and may also result in development of cardiac arrhythmias and syndrome of inappropriate antidiuretic hormone secretion.[17–19]

Because erythromycin and some other macrolide antibiotics inhibit CYP 3A4, the list of potential drug interactions associated with their use is beyond the scope of this review. Erythromycin decreases the metabolism of some benzodiazepine sedative-hypnotic agents, such as alprazolam, triazolam, and midazolam, resulting in a marked increased in somnolence.[20] In addition, erythromycin may reduce the intestinal and hepatic metabolism of cyclosporin, leading to an increase in cyclosporin serum levels.[21]

Rifampin

Rifampin, a rifamycin antibiotic, is a potent enzyme inducer that has been associated with several clinically significant drug interactions.[22] Through enzyme induction of hepatic CYP enzymes, such as CYP 3A4, rifampin markedly accelerates the metabolism of several other drugs, including estrogen, corticosteroids, cyclosporin, and azole antifungal agents, such as ketoconazole and itraconazole.[3–5,12,15,16,23] For example, oral contraceptive failure has been reported because of administration of rifampin in women using oral contraceptive agents.[15,23] Treatment failure has also been reported with other agents after administration of rifampin, including corticosteroids and antifungal agents.[22,23] Before prescribing rifampin, it is important that the clinician consider potential drug interactions secondary to enzyme induction produced by rifampin.

OTHER INTERACTIONS OF POTENTIAL CLINICAL SIGNIFICANCE
Trimethoprim/Sulfamethoxazole

Trimethoprim/sulfamethoxazole (TMP-sulfa), or trimethoprim alone, has been reported to increase the risk for hematologic toxicity in patients receiving methotrexate.[24] Coadministration is best avoided.

SUMMARY

Oral antibiotics are commonly prescribed by dermatologists in clinical practice. When prescribing an oral antibiotic, as with other systemic medications, it is important to consider potential interactions with other drugs, including over-the-counter medications. The most common drug interaction mechanisms that may lead to clinically significant sequelae are inhibition of GI drug absorption and alterations in drug metabolism. Tetracycline and quinolones undergo chelation interactions with many metal ions found in antacids and mineral supplements. Some macrolides, such as erythromycin, inhibit the hepatic metabolism of many other drugs, increasing the risk for toxicity. Rifampin increases the metabolism of many other drugs, thus predisposing to treatment failure. Drug interactions can only be averted if their potential is understood and recognized in advance.

REFERENCES

1. Leyden JJ, Del Rosso JQ, Webster GF. Clinical considerations in the treatment of acne vulgaris and other inflammatory skin disorders: focus on antibiotic resistance. Cutis 2007;79(Suppl 6):9–25.
2. Del Rosso JQ, Leyden JJ, Thiboutot D, et al. Antibiotic use in acne vulgaris and rosacea: clinical considerations and resistance issues of significance to dermatologists. Cutis 2008;82(Suppl 2):5–12.
3. Michalets E. Update: clinically significant cytochrome P450 drug interactions. Pharmacotherapy 1998;18:84–112.
4. Anderson W, Feingold D. Adverse drug interactions clinically important for the dermatologist. Arch Dermatol 1995;131:468–73.
5. Barranco VP. Clinically significant drug interactions in dermatology. J Am Acad Dermatol 1998;38:599–612.
6. Seidlik PH, Olson SC, Yang BB, et al. Erythromycin coadministration increases plasma atorvastatin concentrations. Pharm Res 1996;13(Suppl 9):S437.
7. Schentag JJ, Watson WA, Nix DE, et al. Time dependent interactions between antacids and quinolone antibiotics. Clin Pharmacol Ther 1988;43:135.

8. Leyden JJ. Absorption of minocycline hydrochloride and tetracycline hydrochloride: effects of food, milk, and iron. J Am Acad Dermatol 1985;12:308–12.

9. Ericsson CD, Feldman S, Pickering LK, et al. Influence of subsalicylate bismuth on absorption of doxycycline. JAMA 1982;247:2266–7.

10. Neuvonen PJ, Gothoni G, Hackman R, et al. Interference of iron with the absorption of tetracyclines in man. Br Med J 1970;4:532–5.

11. Nix DE, Watson WA, Lener ME, et al. Effects of aluminum and magnesium antacids and ranitidine on the absorption of ciprofloxacin. Clin Pharmacol Ther 1989;46:700–5.

12. Singer MI, Shapiro LE, Shear NH. Cytochrome P450 3A: interactions with dermatologic therapies. J Am Acad Dermatol 1997;37:765–71.

13. Gupta AK, Katz HI, Shear NH. Drug interactions with itraconazole, fluconazole, and terbinafine and their management. J Am Acad Dermatol 1999;41: 237–49.

14. Neuvonen PJ, Jalava KM. Itraconazole drastically increases plasma concentrations of lovastatin and lovastatin acid. Clin Pharmacol Ther 1996;60:54–61.

15. Skolnick JL, Stoler BS, Katz DB, et al. Rifampicin, oral contraceptives, and pregnancy. JAMA 1976; 236:1382.

16. Bolt HM, Kappus H, Bolt M. Effect of rifampicin treatment on the metabolism of oestradiol and 17-alpha ethinyl oestradiol by human liver microsomes. Eur J Clin Pharmacol 1975;8:301–7.

17. Wong YY, Ludden TM, Bell RD. Effect of erythromycin on carbamazepine kinetics. Drug Intell Clin Pharm 1982;16:484–5.

18. Hedrick R, Williams F, Morin R, et al. Carbamazepine-erythromycin interaction leading to carbamazepine toxicity in four epileptic children. Ther Drug Monit 1983;5:405–7.

19. Zitelli BJ, Howrie DL, Altman H, et al. Erythromycin-induced drug interactions. Clin Pediatr 1987;26: 117–9.

20. Phillips JP, Antal EJ, Smith RB. A pharmacokinetic interaction between erythromycin and triazolam. J Clin Psychopharmacol 1986;6:297–9.

21. Jensen CWB, Flechner SM, Van Buren CT, et al. Exacerbation of cyclosporin toxicity by concomitant administration of erythromycin. Transplantation 1987;43:263–70.

22. Zhou SF. Drugs behave as substrates, inhibitors and inducers of human cytochrome P450 3A4. Curr Drug Metab 2008;9:310–22.

23. Baciewicz AM, Chrisman CR, Finch CK, et al. Update on rifampin and rifabutin drug interactions. Am J Med Sci 2008;335:126–36.

24. Govert JA, Patton S, Fine RL. Pancytopenia from using trimethoprim and methotrexate. Ann Intern Med 1992;117:877–8.

Index

Note: Page numbers of article titles are in **boldface** type.

Dermatol Clin 27 (2009) 95–98
doi:10.1016/S0733-8635(08)00094-6

Moving?

Make sure your subscription moves with you!

To notify us of your new address, find your **Clinics Account Number** (located on your mailing label above your name), and contact customer service at:

E-mail: elspcs@elsevier.com

800-654-2452 (subscribers in the U.S. & Canada)
314-453-7041 (subscribers outside of the U.S. & Canada)

Fax number: 314-523-5170

Elsevier Periodicals Customer Service
11830 Westline Industrial Drive
St. Louis, MO 63146

*To ensure uninterrupted delivery of your subscription, please notify us at least 4 weeks in advance of move.